OXFORD MEDICAL P

Lung Can

THE FACTS

ALSO PUBLISHED BY OXFORD UNIVERSITY PRESS

Ageing: the facts
(second edition)
Nicholas Coni, William Davison,
and Stephen Webster

Alcoholism: the facts
(second edition)
Donald W. Goodwin

Allergy: the facts
Robert Davies and Susan Ollier

**Arthritis and rheumatism:
the facts** (second edition)
J. T. Scott

Autism: the facts
Simon Baron-Cohen and
Patrick Bolton

Back pain: the facts
(third edition)
Malcolm I. V. Jayson

Bowel cancer: the facts
John M. A. Northover and
Joel D. Kettner

Contraception: the facts
(second edition)
Peter Bromwich and
Tony Parsons

**Coronary heart disease:
the facts** (second edition)
Desmond Julian and
Claire Marley

Cystic fibrosis: the facts
(second edition)
Ann Harris and Maurice Super

Deafness: the facts
Andrew P. Freeland

Down syndrome: the facts
Mark Selikowitz

**Dyslexia and other learning
difficulties: the facts**
Mark Selikowitz

Eating disorders: the facts
(third edition) Suzanne Abraham
and Derek Llewellyn-Jones

Head injury: the facts
Dorothy Gronwall, Philip
Wrightson, and Peter Waddell

Healthy skin: the facts
Rona M. MacKie

Kidney disease: the facts
(second edition)
Stewart Cameron

**Liver disease and gallstones:
the facts** (second edition)
Alan G. Johnson and
David R. Triger

Lung cancer: the facts
(second edition)
Chris Williams

Multiple sclerosis: the facts
(third edition)
Bryan Matthews

**Obsessive–compulsive disorder:
the facts**
Padmal de Silva and
Stanley Rachman

Parkinson's disease: the facts
(second edition)
Gerald Stern and Andrew Lees

Pre-eclampsia: the facts
Chris Redman and Isabel Walker

Thyroid disease: the facts
(second edition) R. I. S. Bayliss
and W. M. G. Tunbridge

Lung Cancer

THE FACTS
Second Edition

CHRIS WILLIAMS
Cancer Research Campaign,
Wessex Regional Medical Oncology Unit
University of Southampton

OXFORD NEW YORK TOKYO
OXFORD UNIVERSITY PRESS

Oxford University Press, Walton Street, Oxford OX2 6DP
Oxford New York Toronto
Delhi Bombay Calcutta Madras Karachi
Kuala Lumpur Singapore Hong Kong Tokyo
Nairobi Dar es Salaam Cape Town
Melbourne Auckland Madrid
and associated companies in
Berlin Ibadan

Oxford is a trade mark of Oxford University Press

Published in the United States
by Oxford University Press Inc., New York

© *C. J. Williams, 1992*
First published 1984
Second edition 1992
Reprinted 1993

All rights reserved. No part of this publication may be reproduced,
stored in a retrieval system, or transmitted, in any form or by any means,
electronic, mechanical, photocopying, recording, or otherwise, without
the prior permission of Oxford University Press

This book is sold subject to the condition that it shall not, by way
of trade or otherwise, be lent, re-sold, hired out, or otherwise circulated
without the publisher's prior consent in any form of binding or cover
other than that in which it is published and without a similar condition
including this condition being imposed on the subsequent purchaser

A catalogue record for this book is available from the British Library

Library of Congress Cataloging in Publication Data
Williams, C. J. (Christopher John Hacon)
Lung cancer : the facts / Chris Williams. - 2nd ed.
Includes bibliographical references and index.
1. Lungs—Cancer. I. Title. II. Series.
[DNLM: 1. Lung Neoplasms—popular works. WF 658 W722L]
RC280.L8W55 1992   616.99'424—dc20   91-46202
ISBN 0-19-262251-X
ISBN 0-19-262250-1 (pbk.)

Printed and bound in Great Britain
by Biddles Ltd
Guildford and King's Lynn

Contents

Part 1 About lung cancer	1
1. What is lung cancer?	3
2. Who gets lung cancer?	10
3. What causes lung cancer?	14
4. Stopping smoking	24
5. How is lung cancer diagnosed?	29
6. Tests used to stage lung cancer	38
Part 2 Treatment	47
7. Treatment of non-small-cell cancer	49
8. Treatment of small-cell lung cancer	67
9. Treatment of other lung tumours	74
10. Other methods of treatment	78
11. Treatment of the symptoms and complications of lung cancer	82
12. Talking about lung cancer	98
Part 3 The future	101
13. Clinical trials	103
14. Future prospects in lung cancer	106
15. The new biology	111
Further reading	118
Appendix: Sources of help	120
Glossary	142
Index	145

Part 1 About lung cancer

1
What is lung cancer?

We have all heard about lung cancer, but most of us have only a rudimentary idea of the disease and its treatment, and even this is coloured by our own emotional reaction to the idea of cancer itself. The aim of this book, therefore, is to give, in a clear and simple way, quite detailed information about all aspects of this type of cancer, though with a stress on the practical side of its treatment.

Before we can answer the question 'what is lung cancer?' we need to know what cancer itself is. The body is made up of millions of individual cells, most of which are capable of dividing and reproducing themselves so that the body can grow and, if injured, repair itself. The division of cells to form new cells is carefully controlled in the normal body, much as a car's speed is controlled by the brake and accelerator, so that extra, unwanted cells are not produced. A cut, for instance, will heal because the cells in the skin respond to a signal telling them to divide to form new cells, which fill in the injured area. However, as soon as the skin has healed, the cells appear to respond to another signal that tells them it is time to stop dividing. The nature of the signals that stop and start cells dividing is not fully understood and is a major area of biological research. Very occasionally a cell may develop in which the mechanisms controlling cell divisions are defective. Such a new cell may be permanently 'switched on' and continue to divide, or simply cannot respond to the normal signal telling it to brake and stop dividing. If this cell goes on dividing the new cells it produces are likely to lack the normal mechanisms controlling cell division, and may also carry on growing unchecked. Eventually these cells will form a cancer.

Initially the cells pile up haphazardly where they start to grow, but they may also spread to other parts of the body by invading local tissues or through the blood vessels or lymphatic system (a network of fine vessels joining the lymph nodes; see p. 33). The characteristics by which we recognize cancer are therefore:

- uncontrolled growth, which is unresponsive to the normal signals that tell cells when to divide and when not to;

- a tendency to invade local tissues;
- a tendency to spread (metastasize) widely in the body.

The development of a cancer is, in reality, very much more complex and cells often undergo changes so that they are clearly abnormal but not yet cancerous (a premalignant stage) before they eventually become a malignant tumour. Many lung cancers go through this cycle and it is often possible to see these precancerous cells in the lining of the airways in the lung. Most of them do not undergo further changes, but some may, and these cells form a cancer. The development of lung cancer is not well understood but findings in animals and in human lung tissue suggest that the sequence of events described in Table 1 takes place in one particular type of lung cancer (squamous cancer; see p. 6):

The development of the other major types of lung cancer (see below) is much less well known but may well involve a similar sequence of premalignant changes.

Table 1. Sequence of events in the development of squamous lung cancer

1. There is inflammation of cells lining the airways into the lung, with loss of the lining cells (ciliated cells) that clear secretions from the airways, and overgrowth and piling up of deeper cells.

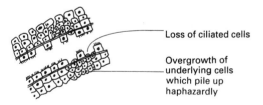

Loss of ciliated cells

Overgrowth of underlying cells which pile up haphazardly

2. The normal plump lining cells (columnar cells) of the airways change to a flatter type (squamous cells). This is referred to as metaplasia.

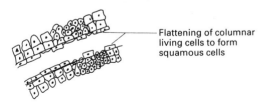

Flattening of columnar living cells to form squamous cells

What is lung cancer?

3. Increasingly abnormal metaplastic cells (now called dysplastic cells) appear. These changes are found in over 90 per cent of active smokers, in 6 per cent of people who have stopped smoking for more than 5 years, and only in 1 per cent of non-smokers. They are, therefore, obviously reversible and do not mean that cancer is inevitable when dysplastic changes have developed.

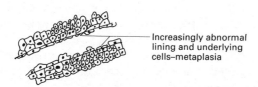

Increasingly abnormal lining and underlying cells—metaplasia

4. The next stage is called 'cancer *in situ*' (a small cancer that has not invaded or spread). This starts somewhere in the dysplastic area and may be several centimetres long and occupy the width of the lining of the airway. Cancer *in situ* is seen in the lungs of 1 in 20 heavy smokers.

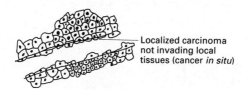

Localized carcinoma not invading local tissues (cancer *in situ*)

5. The small cancer *in situ* may then turn into an invasive cancer. The events that trigger the change from cancer *in situ* to a malignant tumour are not known. When the tumour starts to invade the nearby lung, lymph nodes, and other parts of the body it is regarded as a malignant lung cancer.

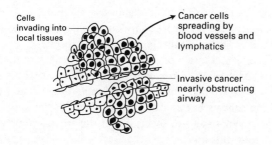

Cells invading into local tissues

Cancer cells spreading by blood vessels and lymphatics

Invasive cancer nearly obstructing airway

6 **Lung cancer: the facts**

TYPES OF LUNG CANCER

Lung cancer is not one disease. There are, in fact, several kinds of cancer that can develop in the lungs (Table 2) and each can be recognized by its appearance when looked at through a microscope. Each type tends to behave in a different manner and there is evidence that they may be caused in different ways. Although these differences are important for our future understanding of the disease they are not, at present, of much help to doctors when they are deciding on treatment. Because of this, the common lung cancers have been divided into two major groups for the purposes of choosing treatment (Table 2):

(1) small-cell lung cancer;
(2) non-small-cell lung cancer.

Table 2. The main types of lung cancer

Type of cancer		Estimated incidence (%)
Squamous carcinoma	Collectively referred	34
Adenocarcinoma	to as non-small-cell	25
Large-cell carcinoma	carcinoma	15
Small-cell carcinoma		25
Mesothelioma		1

Mesothelioma, a tumour of the lining around the lungs (the pleura), differs greatly from these two more common lung cancers and is treated in a different way. It forms a third group of lung cancer.

There are also several rare types of cancer that can start in the lungs; these are discussed briefly in Chapter 9. Many tumours that develop in other parts of the body may spread to the lungs; these should not be regarded as lung cancers but as secondary tumours in the lung. These tumours are treated not as lung cancers, but as the original tumour; they are not discussed in this book.

What is lung cancer?

CHARACTERISTICS OF THE MAIN TYPES OF LUNG CANCER

SQUAMOUS LUNG CANCER

This is the most common kind of cancer in the lungs and has a characteristic appearance when looked at through a microscope. It is called squamous carcinoma because its cells resemble a type of flat-surfaced cell called a squamous cell. The tumour cells produce keratin, a substance normally found in skin and hair, and which can be seen in the tumour. It is very much more common in smokers, develops in the major airways (the large bronchi; see Fig. 8, p. 31), and spreads by invading the local tissues, from where it spreads to lymph nodes and into the bloodstream. Extensive premalignant dysplastic changes and metaplasia (see p. 4) often accompany this tumour.

ADENOCARCINOMA

This tumour is derived from glandular tissue and can often be recognized by its attempt to form new glands. Adenocarcinomas usually develop beneath the lining (mucosa) of the airways, which can make them more difficult to diagnose. Many start in the periphery of the lung rather than in the centre of the chest and they may be easier to remove surgically because of this. Smoking does not seem to predispose this particular type of lung cancer. The tumour spreads in the airways and to lymph nodes, and eventually in the blood. Bronchioloalveolar carcinoma, an unusual tumour in which there is often widespread involvement in both lungs, is probably a special type of adenocarcinoma.

LARGE-CELL CARCINOMA

As might be expected, the cells in this tumour are rather larger than in other types. They show no attempt to form recognizable structures, like glands, and neither do they produce keratin. These tumours are usually found in smokers and may develop in the central or peripheral part of the lungs. They spread within the airways, to the lymph glands, and by the bloodstream.

8 Lung cancer: the facts

SMALL-CELL CARCINOMA

The cells of this tumour are small and fragile. They are often divided into different groups by their shape and some are called 'oat-cell', because of their similarity to oat grains. They nearly always develop in smokers, usually in the central part of the lung, and spread to the lymph glands and bloodstream early in the development of the cancer. These tumours are thought to develop from a special type of cell concerned with making chemical messengers (hormones) and, in support of this, special structures that produce the hormones (neurosecretory granules) can be seen in the cancer cells under the high magnification of an electron microscope. The rate of growth of these tumours is greater than that of the other main types of lung cancer and tumour cells have often spread to distant parts of the body by the time the diagnosis is made.

A carcinoid tumour (see p. 76) is a rare type of lung cancer that also develops from the special hormone-producing cells. It generally has a much less malignant course than small-cell lung cancer.

MESOTHELIOMA

This is a tumour of the lining or membrane (pleura) surrounding the lung and separating it from the chest wall (see Fig. 8, p. 31). Most tumours occur after exposure to asbestos and they may also develop in the lining of the abdominal cavity—the peritoneum. They frequently cause fluid to accumulate between the lung and chest wall (a pleural effusion). Although they have a characteristic appearance under a microscope, on a chest X-ray they are sometimes difficult to diagnose or to distinguish from a cancer that has spread from other parts of the body.

TUMOUR GRADE

This is a measure of the degree of normality of the individual tumour cells and of structures that they form when looked at using a microscope. For instance, an adenocarcinoma that forms easily-recognized glands is said to be of a good grade, or well-differentiated. Poor-grade tumours have very abnormal-looking cells and few recognizable normal structures and, because of this, it can be difficult to tell a poorly differentiated adenocarcinoma or squamous carcinoma from a large-cell tumour.

So, although lung cancers are divided into different types, it is not always easy to be sure into which group an individual cancer falls. The

What is lung cancer?

situation is further complicated by some cases in which there is a mixture of more than one of the main kinds of tumour.

SPECIAL TESTS

MONOCLONAL ANTIBODIES

Antibodies are proteins produced in the body which have the ability to recognize specific structures on other cells or proteins. We are now able to make antibodies in the laboratory which recognize one particular structure; these are called monoclonal antibodies. By attaching a marker to the monoclonal antibody, it is possible to show using a microscope or other techniques whether the monoclonal antibody is sticking preferentially to tumour cells or not. Monoclonal antibodies can be used to differentiate between tumours that are derived from different tissues but which look very similar under the microscope. For instance, small-cell lung cancer may sometimes look like the cells seen in cancer of the lymph glands—lymphoma. Monoclonal antibodies can quickly and clearly substantiate whether the tumour was derived from a lymph gland or the lung since we have developed monoclonals specific for structures on lymphoma cells and lung cancers.

ELECTRON MICROSCOPY

Electron microscopy may show features that help the pathologist to decide on the type of tumour he or she is dealing with. Similarly, a number of biochemical markers have been identified that can help in sorting out small-cell tumours from the other common types of lung cancer. However, the situation has become more complicated since the discovery that some of the so-called non-small-cell cancers share biochemical markers with small-cell tumours, and respond to treatment more like small-cell cancer.

The identification of some of the genes that control normal and malignant cell division (oncogenes) has resulted in studies of the expression of these oncogenes in individual cancers (see Chapter 15). There is evidence that abnormal expression of some oncogenes in lung cancer is associated with a worse prognosis.

A wide variety of normal and abnormal hormones are produced by lung cancer cells, especially small-cell lung cancer cells. These hormones are being studied to see if they correlate with prognosis or whether their presence can be manipulated for therapeutic benefit.

2
Who gets lung cancer?

Cancer of the lung is primarily a disease of well-developed affluent countries and studies of deaths from cancer in different parts of the world show that people living in the United Kingdom have the highest risk of developing lung cancer. Higher rates are seen in the industrialized countries than in the developing countries, and Nigeria is at the bottom of the world lung cancer league (Fig. 1). The rest of this chapter is mainly concerned with industrialized countries, as these have been studied more closely.

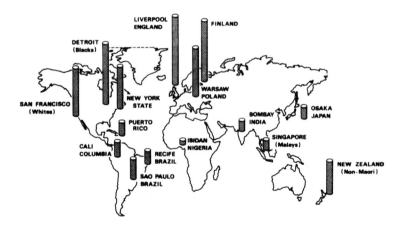

Fig. 1 The risk of developing lung cancer in different parts of the world (1966-7).

Many more men than women develop lung cancer and it is a disease that is most common in those in their 60s and 70s.

The increase in the incidence of death from lung cancer since the turn of the century has been phenomenal; indeed, lung cancer was regarded as very rare until this century. The rate of increase peaked for men in the late 1970s and is now falling but the number of deaths from lung cancer continues to increase alarmingly in women. The importance of lung cancer as a cause of death can be seen in Figure 2. This three-dimensional graph shows the proportion of deaths due to lung cancer out of all deaths

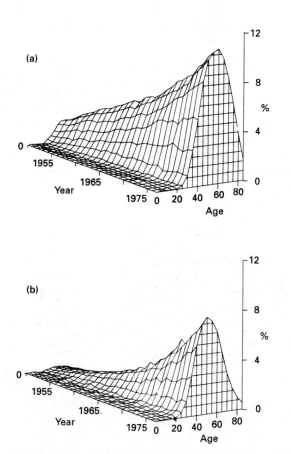

Fig. 2 Deaths from lung cancer in (a) men and (b) women in the United States (1950–77).

in the United States for the years 1950–77. The first graph (a), for men, shows that the highest rate of lung cancer deaths is in the age group 60–64 years and that the proportion of patients in this age group dying from lung cancer has risen from less than 4 per cent in 1950 to nearly

12   Lung cancer: the facts

11 per cent of all deaths in 1977. Women, in graph (b), seem to die from lung cancer at an earlier age (50–54 years) and the proportion has risen from less than 2 per cent to nearly 8 per cent of all deaths in this age group. Lung cancer, therefore, kills nearly 1 in 10 people in their 60s dying in the United States. It is by far the most common cancer in men and is poised to overtake breast cancer as the most common cancer in women (it has just done so in the west of Scotland). In crude terms, 40 000 people in the United Kingdom and 140 000 people in the United States died from lung cancer in 1990.

The next chapter discusses in more detail the possible causes of lung cancer but there are some factors that allow us to pick out those people at highest risk. The profile of someone at highest risk includes:

- living in a westernized society;
- being a man;
- being a smoker;
- being aged 60 or more;
- living in an urban environment.

Exposure to certain cancer-causing chemicals or substances (carcinogens) at work can also result in lung cancer (Table 3). Of course, not everyone who works in these industries is exposed to carcinogens, but it is very important that any safety regulations are enforced and obeyed. The problems associated with the asbestos industry illustrate how difficult it is to avoid needless exposure to carcinogens. However, over the years some companies have failed to comply with safety procedures and their workers have often ignored advice on precautions: and this happened despite our knowledge of some of the risks of asbestos.

We need to know more about the cancer risks of various jobs and how to reduce these risks (including, as a last resort, banning some carcinogens). One of the main problems is the long time, know as the latent period, between exposure to the cancer-causing substance and the eventual development of a malignant tumour. This may be as long as 20 or more years and makes it difficult for workers and companies to take the risks seriously. Many people have died of cancer caused by a very short period of asbestos exposure 30 or 40 years earlier—the risks are only appreciated when it is too late.

Anyone who may be exposed to carcinogens, such as asbestos, at work should try to stop smoking, as cigarettes seem to work together with the carcinogen and the two greatly increase the risk of lung cancer.

Occasionally there may be a tendency for a family to be at high risk of developing cancer, and this may include cancers of the lung. However,

Who gets lung cancer?

Table 3. Jobs that carry an increased risk of lung cancer*

Cancer-causing substance	Job
Arsenic	Oil refining, smelting, mining, using insecticides, tanning, working in the chemical industry
Chromium	Glassmaking, potting, acetylene and aniline manufacturing, bleaching, battery making
Iron oxide	Iron founding, iron ore mining, silver finishing, metal grinding and polishing
Asbestos	Asbestos milling and manufacture, working with insulation, ship yard working, brake and clutch repairing, asbestos mining
Petroleum products and oils	Working in contact with lubricating oils, paraffins or wax oils or coke and rubber
Coal tar and products of	Working with asphalt, tar, and pitch, working in the coke-gas industry, working as a stoker, chimney sweep, mining
Bis(chloromethyl) ether and mustard gas	Working in the chemical industry
Radiation	Working in the radiation industry, medicine, radiology

* Remember that not everyone in these industries is exposed to carcinogens. If you are concerned consult your company's doctor or your trade union.

only those family members who smoke or who are exposed to carcinogens are likely to get cancer.

No relationship between lung cancer and alcohol or drugs has been shown and air pollution has never been conclusively shown to cause cancer, although those who live in urban areas with more pollution seem to have a higher risk. Radon gas has recently been implicated as a potential cause of lung cancer. This radioactive gas is released from the ground into the foundations of some buildings and, if the buildings are well insulated, the gas may reach relatively high concentrations. It is known that this gas can cause lung cancer in working miners and it is being investigated to see if it is a hazard in the home and workplace. Radon levels vary greatly from one part of the country to another and high levels are only found in certain locations.

3
What causes lung cancer?

Lung cancer is a disease of the twentieth century, indeed, in 1912 a well-known US doctor wrote: 'primary cancers of the lung are among the rarest forms of the disease'. Medical students of that day hardly saw a single case during their training; unfortunately this is far from the case now. Lung cancer is now the most common tumour in the developed world and accounts for nearly half of all cancer deaths in men. Although the incidence of lung cancer has increased in all countries, the United Kingdom has led the trend and has the highest rates for this tumour in the world. Any explanation of the cause of lung cancer must, therefore, take into account the huge increase in the incidence of the cancer this century: an increase that has occurred while the death rates from several other tumours have fallen (Fig. 3). It should also account for the geo-

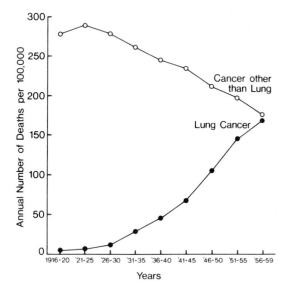

Fig. 3 Death rate for lung cancer and other types of cancer in middle-aged men between 1916 and 1959. ●────● lung cancer; ○────○ cancer other than lung cancer.

graphical distribution of the tumour. These factors strongly suggest an environmental cause and rule out genetic factors, because the genetic make up of the population could not change so quickly. Lung cancer has been blamed on many factors, but by far the most important is smoking.

SMOKING

The habit of smoking, chewing, or taking tobacco as snuff has been common in Europe for over 400 years, so why should there be a sudden increase in lung cancer deaths? Although tobacco has been used for a long time, it is only in the past hundred years that cigarette smoking has been common, and only in this century that tobacco has become mild enough to be inhaled into the lungs. Apparently it is the inhalation of tobacco smoke deep into the lungs that causes lung cancer, and this is a relatively recent habit.

Cigarette smoking as we know it started during the Crimean War (1853-6), and the first major boost in tobacco sales came with the First World War (Fig. 4). Cigarettes were lauded for their ability to induce tranquility and to relieve depression, thirst, and hunger, and every effort was made to ensure that front-line troops received cigarettes—they were even described by one General as being: 'as indispensable as the daily ration'.

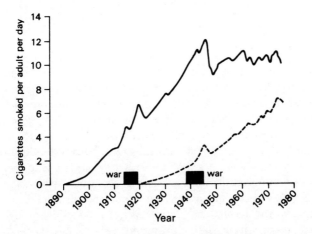

Fig. 4 Consumption of tobacco in the United Kingdom between 1890 and 1975. ——— men; ------- women.

16 Lung cancer: the facts

Following the First World War cigarette sales fell, but intensive advertising and the handing out of free 'starter' packs ensured that more and more men, and then women, became smokers. By the 1930s the majority of the population in the United Kingdom were smokers and the trend towards increased smoking continued. At this time several reports linking smoking and deaths from lung cancer were published in Germany and the United States. However, the number of patients involved were relatively small and the evidence was ignored. The onset of the Second World War stopped further investigation of the risks of cigarette smoking and sales rose even further. Advertising even continued in American medical journals, encouraging doctors with slogans such as: 'the thoughtful physician sends cigarettes to his friends and patients overseas.' Smoking was accepted as socially desirable and few doctors had any qualms about its safety.

INVESTIGATION OF THE LINK BETWEEN SMOKING AND LUNG CANCER

After the Second World War, research workers again started to examine the effects of smoking on health. Initially these studies reviewed the smoking habits of a group of patients with lung cancer and compared them with the smoking habits of a similar group of individuals not suffering from lung cancer (a retrospective survey called a case-control study).

Retrospective surveys

At least 30 investigations from 10 countries have shown by retrospective study among patients with lung cancer that there is a higher proportion of heavy smokers than in comparable control groups. Not only have *all* these studies shown the same association, but in general the results from different countries have been very similar.

The method of investigation used is to record answers to questions about smoking habits given by patients with lung cancer and to compare them with those given by matched individuals, usually patients in the same hospital, without lung cancer. Despite scrupulous care in running such surveys the results are always open to the criticism that an unknown bias may have affected the results.

Although much of the criticism of these early studies was successfully refuted, new studies of fit and healthy populations to find the risk of their

What causes lung cancer?

developing lung cancer according to their smoking habit were clearly needed (prospective surveys).

Prospective surveys

Doll and Hill, the researchers who started retrospective studies in the United Kingdom in the 1950s followed these with a prospective study of over 40 000 male doctors. In the United States several groups of workers, including Hammond and Horn, and Dorn, started similar studies with even larger groups.

All of these prospective studies have confirmed the results of the retrospective studies. The results of the eight prospective studies so far conducted are very similar. All eight show a steady increase in the number of deaths from lung cancer with increasing cigarette consumption, and are in close agreement with the retrospective studies. The increase in the number of deaths with the number of cigarettes smoked in three of the largest studies is shown graphically in Figure 5. Although these studies have been criticized on the grounds that none of them was carried out on a strictly random sample of any population, their unanimous finding that the risk of death from lung cancer is closely associated with cigarette smoking, and to a smaller extent with other forms of

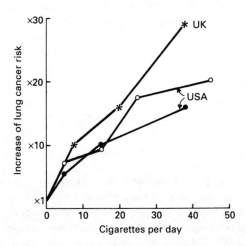

Fig. 5 Relationship between the number of cigarettes smoked and the risk of death from lung cancer in three prospective studies. ●——● and ○--------○ USA; *——* UK.

18   Lung cancer: the facts

smoking, is unchallenged. In addition, post-mortem studies of the lungs of people who have died of diseases other than lung cancer have shown that changes in the lining of the bronchial tubes, of a kind pathologists regard as predisposing to cancer (see p. 4), are common in smokers but seldom seen in non-smokers.

Prospective studies, as well as showing that the risk of developing lung cancer increases with the number of cigarettes smoked (a dose–response effect), also show that the way in which an individual smokes influences the cancer risk. The risk of developing lung cancer is greater in those who inhale the cigarette smoke, who start early in life, who take more puffs on each cigarette, who keep the cigarette in the mouth between puffs, and who relight half-smoked cigarettes. It has also been shown in these studies that men who have switched to filter-tipped cigarettes during the previous 10 years were about 40 per cent less likely to develop lung cancer than men who continued to smoke plain cigarettes. Recent research has shown that cigarettes with a low tar content probably carry a lower risk of lung cancer, although smokers will often circumvent the low tar level by taking more puffs and smoking more cigarettes to keep their nicotine level high.

This prospective and retrospective evidence links smoking and lung cancer deaths with the high incidence of smoking amongst patients with lung cancer. It also shows a clear dose–response effect and further implicates cigarette smoking by the changes in death rate related to subtle variations in the ways in which cigarettes are smoked and the type of cigarettes used.

If cigarette smoking does cause lung cancer, a further powerful piece of evidence confirming this would be a reduction in the death rate from lung cancer of individuals stopping smoking.

REDUCTION OF RISK ON STOPPING SMOKING

All studies have shown a marked reduction of risk of dying from lung cancer in those who have stopped smoking cigarettes compared with those who continue to smoke. This relative reduction is apparent within a few years of stopping. After about 10 years the ex-smoker's risk is only about one-quarter of that of the continuing smoker. The beneficial effect of stopping smoking on lung cancer is best shown in Doll and Hill's study of British doctors, in which over 50 per cent of the smokers stopped during the course of the 20-year study. Between 1954 and 1965

What causes lung cancer? 19

the death rate from lung cancer for these male doctors fell by a staggering 38 per cent, while the rate for all men in the country (whose consumption of tobacco increased slightly) rose by 7 per cent. When the mortality (death rate) of ex-smokers is looked at in relation to the number of years from stopping smoking, a clear benefit for stopping smoking is seen. Many cigarette smokers think that if they have smoked for 20 or more years it is too late to stop smoking because they have already damaged their lungs, but Figure 6 shows that this is just not true.

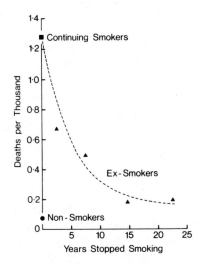

Fig. 6 Relationship between deaths from lung cancer and time since stopping smoking cigarettes.

PASSIVE SMOKING

Non-smoking spouses of smokers have a small but definitely increased risk of developing lung cancer. Much of this information has come from a study of non-smoking wives of Japanese smokers, and it is thought that these women were inhaling the cigarette smoke of their spouse (so-called passive smoking). Someone who does not smoke but whose spouse smokes more than 20 cigarettes a day has twice the risk of lung cancer than if their spouse was a non-smoker. So, as well as removing the unpleasant (for non-smokers) effects of cigarette smoking, prohibition of smoking in public places would reduce the risk of lung cancer for the population as a whole.

20 Lung cancer: the facts

OTHER CAUSES OF LUNG CANCER

AIR POLLUTION

Air pollution, particularly smoke from fossil fuels, appears to increase the risk of lung cancer but its effect is small compared with that of cigarette smoking. It is difficult to estimate the effects of air pollution as those people exposed to air pollution, in industrialized urban areas for instance, are often the people also at risk from excessive smoking and from their jobs. Certain occupations (see Table 3, p. 13) that allow exposure to asbestos dust, chromates, nickel, arsenic, radioactive materials, mustard gas, and the products of coal distillation in the gas industry may result in an increased risk of developing cancer of the lung, particularly if the individuals exposed to these risks are also smokers. However, the number of people at work in such occupations is relatively small and the greatly increased number of deaths from lung cancer cannot be explained by occupational exposure.

VITAMIN A DEFICIENCY

Japanese studies have shown that people deficient in vitamin A (found in green-yellow vegetables) have a higher risk of lung cancer. This vitamin has not been tested to see if supplements to the diet will reduce the risk of lung cancer, although many Western foods already have added vitamins (breakfast cereals for example). Carotenes are currently being tested to see if they can prevent lung cancer developing.

GENETIC FACTORS

It has been suggested that the association between lung cancer and smoking is genetic rather than causal. This hypothesis states that the liability to lung cancer and the desire to smoke cigarettes are inherited genetically and are closely linked. In support of this hypothesis is evidence from studies of twins suggesting a genetic factor in smoking habits and differences between smokers and non-smokers in both physical and psychological characteristics. However, this hypothesis seems an unlikely explanation of the association between lung cancer and smoking because of the failure to account for the great increase in deaths from lung cancer this century.

What causes lung cancer? 21

As a genetically determined disease could not change its frequency in such a short time, and advocates of this hypothesis can only explain the increase in lung cancer on the basis of changes in diagnostic fashion. They postulate that lung cancer has not increased in frequency but that other tumours or diseases were previously diagnosed mistakenly. However, this would not explain the markedly earlier rise in the incidence of lung cancer in men, as changes in diagnostic accuracy would not be confined to one sex. The genetic trait theory also completely fails to account for the fall in the incidence of lung cancer deaths seen in those who stop smoking.

Genetic influences may, however, determine which smokers are likely to develop lung cancer. There is some evidence that cancers, including lung cancer, may be more common in certain families. Only a minority of smokers develop lung cancer and those that do so may have an inherited trait that makes them more susceptible to the cancer-causing factors in cigarette smoke. But even lung-cancer-prone individuals rarely develop the tumour unless they inhale a cancer-producing substance— which for most people is cigarette smoke.

OTHER DISEASES RELATED TO CIGARETTE SMOKING

OTHER CANCERS

Although public awareness of the potential hazards of cigarette smoking is centred on lung cancer, this is only one of many diseases related to smoking. Other types of cancer are more frequent in smokers and a relationship similar to that shown in lung cancer exists. Tumours that are more frequent in smokers include cancer of the mouth, throat, oesophagus (gullet), cervix, pancreas and bladder.

DISEASES OF THE HEART AND BLOOD VESSELS

Increased illness and death from diseases of the heart and blood vessels, despite public concentration on the risks of lung cancer, are more important effects of cigarette smoking than cancer (Table 4). Heart and blood vessel diseases accounted for over half the extra deaths in smokers in Doll's study of British doctors. When coronary heart disease is studied in detail, the incidence of deaths increases with the number of cigarettes smoked at all ages, although it is greatest in young people. In men under

22 Lung cancer: the facts

Table 4. Excess deaths in male smokers by various causes
(British doctors study)

Cause of death	Number of extra (excess) deaths per 100 000 smokers per year
Lung cancer	94 (19%)
Chronic bronchitis and emphysema	47 (10%)
Coronary heart disease	152 (31%)
Other vascular diseases and strokes	100 (21%)
Other diseases	92 (19%)
Total	485 (100%)

45 years of age the death rate per 100 000 was 7 for non-smokers and
104 for those who smoked more than 25 cigarettes per day. Although
the mechanism of the association is unknown, evidence suggests that the
inhalation of carbon monoxide and nicotine may be contributory factors.

Early reports have suggested that the introduction of filter-tipped
cigarettes (which probably reduce the incidence of lung cancer) may
result in high blood levels of carbon monoxide and potentially increase
the incidence of cardiovascular disease.

The effect of smoking on lung cancer is reversible, and this is also true
for cardiovascular disease. In the British doctors' study the death rate
from coronary heart disease in men under 65 years fell steadily throughout the study; in older men there was little change. When the death rate
is studied by smoking habit and the time from stopping smoking it is
found that for both light and heavy smokers it takes about 10–15 years
for the risk from coronary heart disease to fall to that of non-smokers.

BRONCHITIS AND EMPHYSEMA

Chronic bronchitis and emphysema account for about 10 per cent of the
extra deaths caused by smoking. The incidence of bronchitis has been
falling for the past 40–50 years and the most likely explanation for this is
reduced air pollution, decreasing tar content in cigarettes, and improved
treatment. However, bronchitis and emphysema are clearly related to
cigarette smoking and tests of lung function show impairment, which is
most marked in heavy smokers. The damage caused by smoking in this

What causes lung cancer?

condition is mechanical and stopping smoking does not result in improved lung function, although the rate of deterioration is slowed.

SMOKING IN PREGNANCY

Pregnant women who smoke also put their unborn baby at risk: more stillbirths and small babies who die early are born to smokers than to non-smokers. The babies of women who smoke weigh on average 200 grams (7 oz) less than those of non-smokers. Infants and children whose parents smoke are also more prone to chest infection.

Numerous other illnesses are related to smoking and the dangers of cigarette smoking are clearly not confined to an increased risk of lung cancer.

SUMMARY

1. The risk of death from lung cancer is related to the number of cigarettes smoked and the age of starting, and is reduced by smoking filter-tipped cigarettes. There is a small but significant risk for non-smokers when they regularly inhale cigarette smoke (passive smoking).
2. Giving up smoking reduces the risk of death from lung cancer compared to those who continue to smoke and after 15 years, the risk falls to a level similar to that for non-smokers. For those who cannot stop smoking, filter-tipped low-tar cigarettes may be helpful as long as consumption is not increased by smoking more of each cigarette or increasing the number of cigarettes smoked each day.
3. The incidence of lung cancer is increased by exposure to certain chemicals used in industry.
4. There may be a genetic predisposition to lung cancer, as not all heavy smokers develop cancer. However, individuals predisposed to lung cancer may only develop the tumour on exposure to carcinogens such as cigarette smoke.
5. Smoking also increases the death rate from other diseases. Of these, by far the most important is cardiovascular disease (which causes over half the extra deaths due to smoking). Cigarette smoking is also linked to various other tumours, chronic bronchitis, and emphysema. The risk of cardiovascular disease is reduced by stopping smoking and is similar to that of non-smokers 10–15 years after stopping smoking.
6. Smoking is *by far* the single most important avoidable cause of ill health and death in the Western world.

4
Stopping smoking

The title of this chapter makes it sound as though it is easy to give up smoking, but this is far from true. However, despite the undoubted difficulties, anyone with enough will can give the habit up. The strength of will comes from *your* reason for wanting to stop and, if you do not believe there is sufficient reason, it will be very difficult, if not impossible. So, the first step is deciding if you *really* want to stop, and if so, why? The possible advantages are many and include:

- The risk to your health (see Chapter 3): there is an increased risk of lung cancer, heart disease, chronic bronchitis, other cancers, ulcers, and many other conditions. Although many smokers scoff at the thought, and try to pretend it is scaremongering, the risks are deadly serious. Many life assurance companies now offer reduced premiums for non-smokers, and they only bet on certainties. On average those dying of diseases caused by smoking lose 10–15 years of their life.
- The cost: most smokers would have an extra £10–20 a week to spend.
- You will feel healthier and will be able to breathe more easily when you take exercise.
- You will smell fresher and won't have bad breath and stained teeth and fingers.
- You will have fewer colds and chest infections.
- Your children will be less likely to start smoking.
- You will reduce any risk of chest problems for the rest of your family.

To a non-smoker this list seems compelling; why would anyone give up hundreds of pounds a year and the chance of better health? But many smokers seem blind to the risks, although most would say that health is more important to them than wealth—whilst lighting up their next cigarette. You will have taken the first step in stopping smoking when you really believe that cigarettes are bad for you and that you will also gain positive advantages from stopping. You must believe that the advantages of stopping outweigh the discomforts.

Stopping smoking

There are many ways of approaching the problem and no easy solutions. On page 27 there is a list of organizations who may be able to help you to stop smoking. This may be by providing direct help in clinics that support people stopping smoking or by giving information. It is probably useful to see your GP, who may be able to help you personally or put you in touch with a local group.

Some of the methods, apart from simple moral support while stopping, used to try to help smokers have included:

- *Drug therapy*. This often uses tranquillizers. There is little evidence that this approach is effective and it is probably best avoided.
- *Hypnosis*. Although individual practitioners have claimed high success rates there are no properly controlled trials testing how effective hypnosis is. It seems to suit some smokers, although this may depend on the skill of the therapist and the motivation of the smoker, which may be related to the amount of money the client pays for the treatment.
- *Acupuncture*. Once again, no studies have adequately tested the effectiveness of acupuncture. Some smokers seem to find it helpful.
- *Aversion therapy*. This is usually a form of oversmoking or rapid smoking designed to make smoking so unpleasant that the smoker cannot tolerate any more. There is little evidence that it works for very long, although it may well take away the desire to smoke for a short period.
- *Group therapy*. As an extension to simple supportive therapy, more formal group therapy sessions are being tested by organizations interested in reducing smoking.
- *Placebo*. Some anti-smoking 'drugs' available at chemists are inactive and act as a placebo, providing a prop or encouragement. Dummy cigarettes fall into this category.
- *Nicotine chewing gum*. This is currently being tested but the early results do not seem to be as promising as was hoped. The idea is to use nicotine chewing gum as a way of supplying nicotine to the body without the harmful effects of smoking.

If you decide that you really want to give up smoking, get help and support from your family, doctor, and, if possible, a nearby group. There is no secret method; all the above ways have been found helpful by some and it is a case of choosing a method that seems likely to suit you.

Although there is no easy way, some of the following may ease things for you:

26 Lung cancer: the facts

- Try to find someone who you can stop smoking with. If necessary, get sponsors or make a wager.
- Ask your family to be patient and to support you. Warn them that you may be moody and undergo a temporary personality change.
- Pick a quiet day to stop. Get rid of *all* ashtrays, cigarettes, and lighters the night before.
- STOP smoking. That means no cigarettes at all. Most studies suggest that stopping suddenly is better than gradually reducing your cigarette consumption.
- Try to find something to do at the danger times when you normally had a cigarette—after meals, whilst watching television, etc. As well as these new activities, try to find something to do with your hands.
- If you do crave a cigarette, go and find something else to do. Just sitting worrying about it won't work. Try to find your own distraction. After some weeks the craving will gradually decrease, as will the irritability and lack of concentration that often accompany stopping smoking.
- Learn to relax. Some groups can give help with relaxation exercises, and cassette tapes are available. Hypnosis can be helpful.
- Do not let anyone persuade you that 'one won't hurt'. Part of you will be happy to have a cigarette and the first time you give in could be the end of the road. Friends can often be your worst enemy; you will have to put up with their jokes and temptations. Avoid places, such as pubs, where you are likely to meet such 'friends'.
- Watch what you eat. Do not try to diet at the same time; two stresses at once mean that you are likely to fail at both, but do eat sensibly. Many smokers tend to put on weight when they stop, so avoid excess sugary and fatty foods. Remember that this may be the first time that you have really tasted food for years. Do not worry if you put on some weight—you can always deal with that later.
- Arrange to reward yourself when you reach goals. For instance, after one month without cigarettes you can afford a reward, as you may have saved £2 or more a day.
- Imagine the possible consequences of starting smoking again—think of it as like playing Russian roulette.
- Keep working at it. Stopping smoking is not just a passive process. Keep telling yourself why you are stopping. Find things to do when you need a cigarette. Take exercise. Save the money you would have spent so that you can see it grow. Work together with your family and, if possible, your doctor or a group. Don't relax after a few

Stopping smoking 27

weeks. The only really important factor in stopping is your motivation and reasons; any other help is secondary. To be successful you must need to stop smoking more than you need the next cigarette.

HELPFUL ORGANIZATIONS

These organizations may be able to help or put you in touch with those who can.

ASH (Action on Smoking and Health)
5-11 Mortimer Street
London
W1N 7RH
Tel   071 637 9843

HEC (Health Education Council)
78 New Oxford Street
London
WC1A 1AH
Tel   071 637 1881

SHEG (Scottish Health Education Group)
Health Education Centre
21 Landsdowne Crescent
Edinburgh
EH12 5EH
Tel   031 447 8044

UCF (Ulster Cancer Foundation)
40-42 Eglantine Avenue
Belfast
BT9 6DX
Tel   0232 663281

Contact general cancer organizations (see Appendix) who may be able to give you information and find groups in your area. Talk to your general practitioner, who will probably know what is available locally.

WHY DO PEOPLE START SMOKING?

If everyone knows or has at least heard that smoking is such a bad thing, why do so many young people take up smoking? Most smokers started

28 Lung cancer: the facts

during adolescence, out of curiosity, out of a sense of independence and rebelliousness. Teenagers are more likely to start if their parents or friends smoke and they see the gains as sufficient to overcome the unpleasant side-effects of starting to smoke—indeed conquering them is an apparent sign of being 'grown-up'.

By the age of 10 years, 7 per cent of boys and 2.5 per cent of girls in England are regular smokers. Once established, the habit is maintained by the physical and social pleasures of smoking and the difficulty in stopping. This group of young smokers will continue to be a social influence on their friends to take up the habit and to join them in being 'grown up'. Although they may have heard of the risks of smoking they think 'it couldn't happen to me'—remember that lung cancer is a disease of middle and late life, and is far removed from childhood.

A disturbing recent trend has been the increase in smoking amongst women and young girls; men have been smoking less. Tobacco manufacturers, realizing this, are now producing brands aimed primarily at women. A subtle influence of current advertising is to accentuate the slimness of models and, by inference, the appetite suppression of smoking. Indeed, one brand uses the name of 'Slims'. However, campaigns to reduce smoking may be starting to work as the proportion of the population that smokes has fallen from 50 per cent in 1960 to about 40 per cent in 1980, and continues to fall. Despite this, attempts to dissuade teenagers from smoking often fail, and new ways of approaching the problem are being looked at. We need to persuade young people that not only may it be damaging to their future health but that it is not a 'smart' thing to do. They will only stop the rush to become smokers when the glamour and the fantasy that it is adult to smoke have been destroyed.

5
How is lung cancer diagnosed?

Most cases of lung cancer are only discovered when someone goes to their doctor feeling unwell. However, about 1 in 20 tumours may be found incidentally on a routine chest X-ray.

SYMPTOMS OF THE COMMON TYPES OF LUNG CANCER

Lung cancer in its earliest phase causes no ill effects at all, but as the tumour grows it starts to cause symptoms, usually due to its invasion into the tissue of the lung and airways. To begin with these symptoms are often intermittent and are brought on or worsened by physical exertion. They gradually become more continuous and new problems start to appear. Often, these symptoms seem to be caused by a 'chest infection' that doesn't respond to the usual antibiotics and it is only when a chest X-ray is taken that the cancer is found.

The most important and common symptoms of lung cancer are shown in Figure 7. Many could be caused by any chest disease or infection but a few, such as coughing up blood (known as haemoptysis), are reason for immediate investigation. About two in every five patients have a cough as their first symptom and virtually all have a cough at some stage in the development of the cancer. The cough is usually persistent or intermittently recurrent, often beginning with an ordinary cold or chest infection but continuing long after the signs of the cold are gone. Anyone who has a persistent cough for some weeks should, therefore, see a doctor. It is no good just calling it a 'smoker's cough'; a new and persistent cough needs to be explained.

COUGH

Coughing is caused by stimulation of sensory nerves in the lining of the airways, anywhere from the vocal chords in the voice box (larynx) down

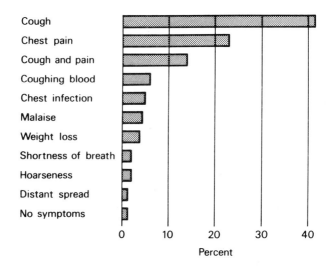

Fig. 7 The frequency of the common symptoms of lung cancer at the time of diagnosis.

to the small airways (bronchi) in the lungs (Fig. 8). It is an involuntary act (reflex), although it can be started voluntarily. Coughing greatly raises the pressure in the chest and the sudden expiration of air is designed to clear away mucous secretions from the lining (mucosa) of the airways. Cancer invading the mucosa of the airways irritates the nerves and starts the cough, which fails to remove the source of irritation—the cancer—and the cough becomes persistent. Any bleeding is very irritant to the lining of the bronchi and will cause blood to be coughed up.

Paroxysms or bouts of coughing may occur if the irritation is bad and cannot be cleared. These paroxysms can be so severe as to crack a rib (a cough fracture) or damage small blood vessels in the lungs. The cough caused by lung cancer is not characteristic but it is often most noticeable at night or first thing in the morning. Later it becomes intermittent throughout the day and paroxysmal. Exertion or deep breathing will often start a coughing fit. Early in the disease the cough is dry but a white mucoid sputum may later be coughed up. If an infection develops this may become a purulent green or yellow and there may be blood in the sputum (haemoptysis) at any stage.

Haemoptysis usually results in some blood streaking of sputum but if (as occasionally happens) a small vein is invaded, fresh blood may be

How is lung cancer diagnosed?

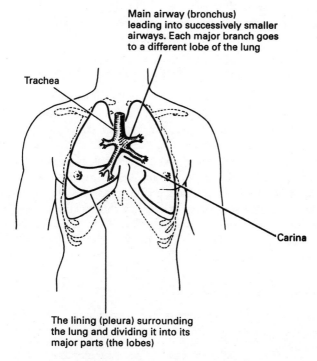

Fig. 8 The anatomy of the chest, major airways, and lungs.

coughed up: it is very rare for there to be severe bleeding. Haemoptysis is a very important symptom that should never be ignored and one in every four people over the age of 40 years who coughs up blood turns out to have lung cancer.

CHEST DISCOMFORT AND PAIN

This is the second most common initial symptom, occurring in about one in five cases, but it develops in nearly all patients at some stage of the illness. Often it is difficult to determine the nature of the pain or discomfort, which can be very variable. The most common description is of fullness and pressure, which is worse in certain positions and on deep breathing or coughing. There may occasionally be a sharp localized pain (pleuritic pain) in the chest on breathing or coughing; this is due to inflammation of the lining over the lung (the pleura).

32   Lung cancer: the facts

Tumours high in the upper part of the lungs (see p. 64) may affect the large nerve roots (brachial plexus) at the base of the neck and can cause progressive pain in the upper chest, shoulder, and upper arm.

CHEST INFECTION AND OBSTRUCTION

Growth of tumour in the larger airways of the lung may gradually result in increasing obstruction of the airway itself. This prevents the normal mucous of the lungs being coughed up and these trapped secretions often become the site for an infection. This causes malaise, chills, fevers, night sweats, and loss of appetite and weight. Infections may respond poorly to conventional antibiotics and, if complete obstruction of the airway ensues, severe shortness of breath, cough, and fevers may develop. The symptoms and their severity depend on how much of the lung is affected.

If the obstruction is incomplete it may cause a wheeze as the air tries to get past the blockage. This is worse on deep breathing, especially after exercise.

SHORTNESS OF BREATH

Shortness of breath is rarely the first symptom of lung cancer, although it is common during the course of the disease. There are various causes which include:

- asthma-like episodes caused by spasm of the airways;
- collapse of the lung caused by obstruction of a major airway (see above);
- infection in the lung;
- fluid between the lung and chest wall (pleural effusion; see p. 85);
- pressure on the major veins around the heart (superior vena caval obstruction; see p. 84), which also causes swelling of the neck veins and face and is made worse by bending forwards;
- collection of fluid in the sac around the heart (pericardial effusion), which restricts the heart's ability to work normally.

HOARSENESS

One of the nerves going to the voice box (larynx) loops down to the root of the left lung in the centre of the chest. A tumour growing in this part of the chest may damage the nerve so that the vocal chords on that side no longer work. This causes a weak, hoarse voice and a typical brassy cough.

How is lung cancer diagnosed? 33

DISTANT SPREAD AND METABOLIC EFFECTS

The tumour may cause general effects—fever, chills, and malaise—because of infection. Less well understood are general symptoms and physical changes that are not directly related to spread of this cancer; these are often called paraneoplastic syndromes. It is presumed that they are caused by hormones or similar substances produced by the tumour or metabolic changes in the body. They include:

- *Skin changes.* These can be very variable but the two most common are a dark rash under the arms or around the neck and upper chest (called acanthosis nigricans) and a skin rash associated with progressive muscle weakness and discomfort (called dermatomyositis).
- *Bone changes.* The most common of these is clubbing—thickening of the finger tips, with typical nail changes. More generalized bone changes (pulmonary hypertrophic osteoarthropathy) can cause painful swellings in the joints of bones of the arms and legs. These symptoms sometimes appear several months before the diagnosis of lung cancer is made.
- *Effects on the nervous system.* All sorts of effects on the nervous system can be seen in patients with lung cancer and these may precede detection of the lung cancer by quite long periods. The most common of these effects is weakness or unsteadiness on walking or getting up from a sitting position (see p. 91).
- *Production of excessive amount of hormones.* Some lung tumours produce normal hormones in excessive amounts and may cause symptoms because of this (see p. 86).

Remember that all of these effects are rather rare and the chances of anyone with a rash or bone problem turning out to have lung cancer is exceedingly small.

SECONDARY OR METASTATIC SPREAD

Tumours of the lung can also spread outside the chest in the lymphatic vessels or in the blood (see p. 4). Symptoms of spread are relatively uncommon as the first evidence of the disease but may develop during the course of the illness. The common sites of spread are:

- Lymph glands in the neck, which become involved in up to half of cases. They can be felt as firm lumps at the root of the neck.

34   Lung cancer: the facts

- Bones, especially the spine, ribs, skull, and limb bones, may become involved in up to 40 per cent of cases.
- Spread to the liver is uncommon at first but may develop in up to half of patients.
- Spread to the brain may occur late in the course of the disease (see p. 89).

TESTS USED TO DIAGNOSE LUNG CANCER

If, after a doctor has heard all about the patient's symptoms and has completed an examination, there is any suspicion of lung cancer, a chest X-ray must be taken immediately. A chest X-ray gives a two-dimensional picture (a photographic negative) of the chest and shows up the different organs by their varying density. Hence, the dense, blood-filled heart is seen as a white area, which contrasts with the dark, air-filled lungs. A tumour, or an area of infection, increases the density of the bit of lung affected and will show up as a denser white area or shadow. By the time lung cancer is suspected the patient's chest X-ray is nearly always abnormal. However, it is impossible for the doctor to know exactly what the abnormal shadow is—it could be infection or many other things—and, even if it is a tumour, an X-ray cannot tell what type it is and the doctor cannot be sure that it started in the lung.

It is, therefore, essential that a bit of the abnormal area or tumour is obtained for examination under a microscope. The test used to do this will depend on exactly where the tumour is.

MICROSCOPIC EXAMINATION

Microscopic examination (cytology) of sputum that has been coughed up may be used to diagnose lung cancer. Cancer cells may be seen in the sputum and, together with a typical chest X-ray, can be used to make the diagnosis of lung cancer. However, many doctors prefer to have the greater accuracy and confidence gained by examining a piece of the tumour itself (a biopsy).

BIOPSY OF A LYMPH NODE

If, on examination, an abnormal lymph gland is found (usually at the root of the neck), it is worth removing this for examination as it gives the best chance of making a firm diagnosis.

How is lung cancer diagnosed? 35

PLEURAL BIOPSY

If there is fluid between the lung and chest wall (pleural effusion), a piece of the pleural lining of the chest may be removed for examination under a microscope. When the fluid is being removed (see p. 85) a special needle is used to cut away a small piece of the pleura. Although this is done after an injection of local anaesthetic it can be uncomfortable and anxious patients should be given a sedative to help reduce any discomfort.

BRONCHOSCOPY

If there are no abnormal lymph glands then a bronchoscopy is done. This means using a tube to look down into the main airways of the lungs (see Fig. 8, p. 31). In the past a metal tube (a rigid bronchoscope) was used but a thin flexible bronchoscope is usually used now. This flexible bronchoscope is made up of optical fibres that can be bent, and that transmit light into the lungs while at the same time allowing the doctor to look into the airways. Rigid bronchoscopes are still used in some situations but flexible bronchoscopes are generally used because they are easier for the patient, don't require a general anaesthetic and because they enable the doctor to see further into the lungs.

When the bronchoscope is in the major airways it is possible to take a small piece of tissue for examination (a biopsy). A brush or sponge is also rubbed against the walls of the airways to pick-up cells that can be examined microscopically. Cells may also be washed out in a small amount of fluid. Using these methods most cancers can be diagnosed with great accuracy.

Bronchoscopy usually only requires admission to hospital as a day case. If a rigid bronchoscope is used, patients are asked to not eat for 12 hours before they come. A short-acting general anaesthetic is given into a vein so that the patient is asleep when the test is done. The bronchoscope is passed in through the patient's mouth whilst their head is tipped back. Before a flexible bronchoscope is used, an injection of a short-acting sedative is given into a vein and an anaesthetic spray is used on the back of the throat. The patient is half awake when this test is done, the thin bronchoscope being passed through a nostril into the back of the throat and then down into the lungs. A few hours after the test the patient may go home, but should not drive because of the sedative or anaesthetic injection they have recently received. Following the test, some patients have a sore throat and a few cough up a little blood.

36   Lung cancer: the facts

ASPIRATION OF LUNG TISSUE

In the case of a suspicious lump in the periphery of the lungs, which is beyond the reach of a bronchoscope, a thin needle may be passed through the skin into the lung itself. Patients are asked to stop breathing for a short time while this is done and a tiny piece of lung tissue is aspirated—sucked out of the lung. The test is done under X-ray control so that the needle can be guided to the suspicious area and experienced doctors have a high rate of success in getting a small piece of lung tissue to make the diagnosis. Leakage of air into the space between the lung and chest wall (pneumothorax; see p. 85) occurs in about 1 in 5 cases but in most it is not serious. Removal of this air (see p. 54) with a drainage tube is sometimes needed, although usually in less than 1 in 10 patients. Occasionally patients cough up some blood after the test has been done.

EXPLORATORY OPERATION

In those few patients (usually with a small single suspicious area in the periphery of the lung) where it is not possible to make a diagnosis using the above tests an exploratory operation (thoracotomy) can be done to examine the lung. As these patients, if it is lung cancer, form the group who are most easily cured by an operation to remove the tumour, it is important not to just wait and see what happens on the X-ray. If it is possible that it could be cancer and all the other tests are unhelpful an operation to remove the lump should be done.

EXPLORATORY OPERATION FOR MICROSCOPIC
EXAMINATION OF LYMPH GLANDS

Where there are enlarged, suspicious glands in the centre of the chest, an exploratory minor operation (mediastinoscopy or mediastinotomy; see p. 40) is undertaken to remove a gland for microscopic examination.

SCREENING FOR LUNG CANCER

Because lung cancer is most curable when it is caught in its earliest stages, attempts have been made to screen healthy people to see if it is possible to pick up lung cancers before they cause symptoms. The idea is that the patients found on screening to have an early cancer will stand a better chance of cure.

How is lung cancer diagnosed? 37

Screening tests have consisted of getting people to cough up sputum samples for cytology (see p. 34) and then having a chest X-ray. The Mayo clinic in the USA has followed two groups of smokers for a number of years. People were allocated, by chance (see p. 105), to either a screening group (chest X-ray and sputum every 4 months) or a non-screening group (no tests). The study found that screening detects malignant tumours at an earlier stage but there was no evidence that those people in the screening group have stood a better chance of being cured. Because of this, large-scale screening has not been recommended. There are, unfortunately, no reliable blood tests that can be used to detect lung cancer at an early stage.

6

Tests used to stage lung cancer

'Staging' is a term used to describe the process of assessing the extent of spread and growth of a malignant tumour. It is done to help select the best treatment and to gain an idea of the patient's outlook. The degree of spread of most cancers is described by a staging system, which defines how big a tumour has grown and how far it has spread, and lung cancer is no exception.

As the approach to treatment is different for small-cell and non-small cell lung cancer, there are separate staging systems for each.

SMALL-CELL CANCER

A very simple system of staging is used for small-cell lung cancer because surgery is much less important in the care of this cancer (Table 5).

Table 5. Staging system for small-cell lung cancer

Limited stage
Disease confined to one side of the chest* and to the draining lymph nodes on that side (including those at the root of the neck)

Extensive stage
Any disease that has spread beyond this (including distant lymph nodes, bone, liver, bone marrow, brain, etc)

---

* Disease may be very extensive within that side of the chest compared with the TNM system (see Table 6).

Chemotherapy is the mainstay of treatment for this tumour and the distinction between limited and extensive disease is more important in understanding the patient's outlook than deciding on the possible use of radiotherapy or surgery, as nearly all patients will be treated primarily with drugs (see p. 67).

Tests used to stage lung cancer

NON-SMALL-CELL CANCER

Surgery is the most important treatment in non-small-cell lung cancer and for this reason the staging system used is much more complicated because it has to give a detailed estimate of the size and distribution of the tumour (Table 6). This type of system is known as a TNM system (T stands for Tumour size, N for lymph Nodes, and M for Metastases—the distant spread of tumour). The importance of such a staging system

Table 6. Simplified staging system for non-small-cell lung cancer *

Primary tumour (T)

T1 Tumour less than 3 cm in diameter, surrounded by normal lung, and not invading the lung more centrally than before the airway leading to that segment of the lung (the lobular bronchus)

T2 Tumour more than 3 cm in diameter, or any size if invading the pleura or associated with some lung collapse or infection. Any such tumour must be more than 2 cm away from the main division of the major airway (carina) (see Fig. 8)

T3 Tumour of any size invading the chest wall, the diaphragm (muscular wall between chest and abdomen), the area around the heart and major blood vessels, or tumour within 2 cm of the carina, or collapse of an entire lung, or a pleural effusion

Draining lymph nodes (N)

N0 No spread to the draining lymph nodes

N1 Spread to the first group of draining lymph nodes

N2 Spread into the lymph nodes in the centre of the chest

Distant metastases (M)

M0 No known metastases

M1 Distant metastases found

---

* The extent of disease estimated by TNM is used to group patients into four stages, with those with the least disease being designated stage 1 and those with the most, stage 4.

is in selecting those patients who will benefit from an operation to remove part or all of the lung and the cancer within it. Clearly only those with a small tumour and with little or no spread to lymph nodes and no spread to other parts of the body will stand a chance of cure with an operation.

40   Lung cancer: the facts

Staging tests

The aims of staging in non-small-cell lung cancer are to define the extent of the primary tumour in the lung and to decide if it has spread to lymph nodes or to distant parts of the body.

Primary tumour (T)

The size and position of the primary tumour (T) is gauged from chest X-rays and by looking directly into the airways to the lungs (bronchoscopy; see p. 00). The chest X-ray will show the size and location of the tumour and whether there is associated lung collapse or infection. Bronchoscopy defines how near the tumour is to the main bronchus.

Lymphatic spread (N)

This can be looked for using several techniques apart from an ordinary chest X-ray.

Computed tomography (CT scan)

This is a new X-ray technique that uses information built-up by a computer rather than an ordinary X-ray film. The computer-produced picture is much better than ordinary X-rays in defining small structures and can show enlarged glands in the centre of the chest. If the glands are enlarged it is highly likely that they contain tumour. However, up to one-quarter of patients whose glands do not appear to be enlarged also turn out to have a tumour, so the test is not absolute. Additional information on the situation and size of the primary cancer in the lung will also be gained from a CT scan.

Mediastinoscopy

Under general anaesthetic a small incision is made at the base of the neck, just above the breast bone (Fig. 9). A special instrument—a mediastinoscope—is passed through the incision into the upper chest. It shines a light into the chest and the doctor can look through it to examine the area around the lungs and heart—the area known as the mediastinum. The doctor can also take a sample (biopsy) of any suspicious areas. This test picks up most abnormal lymph nodes in the area of the chest and it is important to perform mediastinoscopy because an operation to remove the cancer will not be successful if these mediastinal nodes contain cancer.

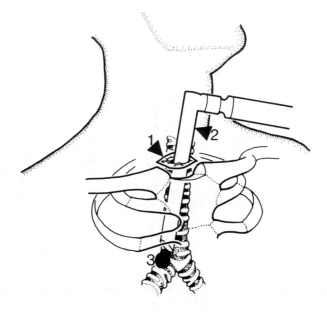

Fig. 9 Mediastinoscopy. A cut is made at the base of the throat (1) and the instrument (2) is passed into the space in the upper chest to look at the glands (3).

Mediastinotomy

This is used as an alternative or if mediastinoscopy fails to give all the information needed. Under general anaesthetic a small operation is done to open the front of the chest, usually between the second and third ribs, on the side where the cancer is growing (Fig. 10). The advantage of this method is that it provides a more direct approach to the mediastinal glands, which can be examined with or without a mediastinoscope. These tests may be used either to make the diagnosis of cancer if no other biopsy can be taken or to see if the mediastinal lymph nodes are involved if an operation is being planned.

Other tests used to look for involvement of lymph nodes

A radioactive isotope (gallium-67) is sometimes used to show-up areas involved with lung cancer. The isotope is concentrated by some lung cancers and shows up as a 'hot spot'—an area of increased uptake—on the image or scan picture. The isotope is given by an injection into a vein and the image is taken using a special radioactive detector, a gamma

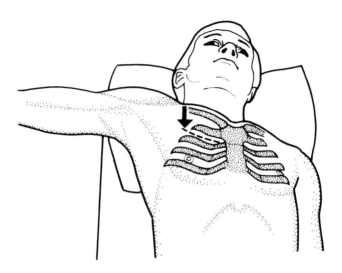

Fig. 10 Typical site for the cut used for mediastinotomy. This may be on either side of the chest.

camera. The test is painless and carries no risk. Special X-rays using dyes that show-up on an ordinary X-ray may also be used to see if there is tumour in the chest. In one of these tests the patient has to swallow some white barium mixture and then has a series of X-rays taken to follow the dye into their stomach. This outlines the oesophagus and shows any enlarged lymph nodes or tumour that may be pressing against or invading the oesophagus. The test is only likely to be done if the patient has difficulty swallowing.

Metastatic disease (M)
This is where the tumour has spread from the lung to other parts of the body. The gallium isotope test mentioned above is occasionally used to look for tumour anywhere in the body, but other tests are usually chosen to look at one part of the body or organ at a time.

The liver
- Blood taken from a vein in the arm is used to see how well the liver is working. However, these tests are not very specific as many factors can affect the way the liver is working. When used together with the tests described below they can, however, add useful information.

Tests used to stage lung cancer 43

- Perhaps the most useful investigation is by ultrasound. In this test, a source of high-frequency sound waves (well beyond what the human ear can hear) is pressed lightly over the part of the body to be examined. The beam of sound waves is bounced back off the various parts of the liver and a computer builds up a picture of the liver according to its varying consistency. Tumours show as areas where there are changes in consistency or density of the liver tissue. This test is very simple, painless, and easily repeated.
- CT scans (see p. 44) can also be used to examine the liver, but are more costly, time-consuming, and may require an injection.
- Radioactive isotopes can be used to produce an image of the liver. An injection of an isotope that is concentrated in the liver is given into a vein in the arm. Tumours fail to take up and concentrate the radioactive isotope and, because of this, show up as a hole or cold area. The image or picture is produced by a gamma camera, the test is painless, without risk but is less sensitive than ultrasound or a CT scan.

The bones

- The most sensitive test is an isotope bone scan. An injection of a radioactive isotope that is absorbed by bones is given into a vein and a picture of the skeleton taken with a gamma camera. Most cancers in bones take up more of the isotope than normal bone and they therefore appear on the picture as a bright hot spot. Occasionally it may fail to take up the isotope and can be seen as a cold spot, or hole. Bone scans often detect tumour before anything can be seen on an X-ray and they are therefore the best way to look at skeleton when staging a cancer. Bone scans detect the amount of bone repair that is going on, so arthritis and injuries often show up. Skilled interpretation of the images produced can usually pick out benign problems from malignant cancers on an abnormal scan.
- A series of X-rays of the main bones in the body—a skeletal survey—can also be used, although cancer only shows up if bone is fairly severely damaged by the tumour. Most cancers thin the affected bone, causing holes, called lytic areas. Occasionally they may cause thickening of the bone, forming blastic or sclerotic areas. Multiple X-rays of bones are not often used now that isotope scans are available, but an X-ray of a limb bone will be taken if an abnormal area is spotted by the bone scan. This is to make sure that there is no

44   Lung cancer: the facts

dangerous thinning of the bone that could lead to a fracture or break.
Any bone that is painful or tender to touch may need to be X-rayed.
- Blood tests may also be useful because a chemical derived from bone
  —alkaline phosphatase—may be present in increased amounts when
  bones are involved with cancer. The amount of calcium in the blood
  is also measured, as high levels will make the patient unwell (see
  p. 88).

The bone marrow

Bone marrow is the soft part in the centre of bones where new blood cells
are made. As lung cancer, and especially small-cell lung cancer, may
spread to the marrow, it is sometimes necessary to take a small sample
for examination under a microscope. This test—a bone marrow aspirate
or biopsy—can be done as an outpatient. An injection of local anaesthetic is given over the bone to be examined, usually the upper part of
the pelvic bone in the lower back or occasionally the breast bone, and a
small needle is passed into the bone. A sample of marrow is then sucked
into a syringe. It is usually uncomfortable at the moment the sample is
sucked out, but most of the pain of the test can be prevented by a local
anaesthetic, and patients who are anxious can be given a sedative
injection. If a biopsy is taken a piece of the marrow is removed using the
same needle.

The brain

Unfortunately some lung tumours do spread to the brain, although it is
unusual for the brain to be involved when cancer is first diagnosed.
Because of this, tests to look for brain metastases are not normally done
unless the patient has symptoms suggesting that there may be a problem
(see p. 89). Several tests may be used to see if the tumour is involving the
brain.

- CT scan is the usual way of looking for tumour in the brain and has
  taken over from many of the more complicated tests used in the past.
  The test is simple and painless, although the injection of X-ray
  contrast dye, which may be used to outline a tumour, will cause a hot
  flush for a few minutes.
- A new type of scanner—a magnetic resonance imaging (MRI)
  scanner—has been developed and is now starting to be used as a
  routine test in some centres. This is another painless test not requiring injections or any unpleasant procedures, although the size
  and complexity of the equipment can be rather daunting. The images

Tests used to stage lung cancer 45

produced can be made from different angles—an advantage over CT imaging, which can only view from one direction.

Other organs

Lung cancer can spread to all sorts of different parts of the body. CT scans are probably the best way to look for such spread in the chest or abdomen. Routine staging tests do not, however, usually include such an extensive search. The number and type of staging tests varies from hospital to hospital and depends on the type of tumour found. The common staging tests for non-small-cell and small-cell cancer are shown in Tables 7 and 8. It should be remembered that, just because the tests are being done, it does not mean there is spread to that organ or even that the doctor suspects that it is likely.

Table 7. Staging tests prior to treatment in non-small-cell lung cancer (appropriate patients will be selected to have some of these tests)

All patients
Physical examination
Chest X-ray
Blood tests
Bronchoscopy
Biopsy of a gland or obvious tumour mass if present

Patients in whom an operation is possible
CT scan of schest
Mediastinoscopy *or* medisatinotomy
Needle biopsy of the tumour in selected patients
Lung function tests
Ultrasound or CT scan of liver
Isotope bone scan

Table 8. Staging tests prior to treatment in small-cell lung cancer

Chest X-ray
Blood tests
Bronchoscopy
Bone marrow (in some hospitals)
Ultrasound or CT examination of the liver
Isotope bone scan

Part 2 Treatment

There are different types of lung cancer and a number of treatments can be used alone or together. Anyone with lung cancer is, of course, hoping for a cure, but unfortunately this is only possible in those who have the smallest amount of disease. Every effort is made to identify the patients who can be cured, and treatment is decided partly on what was found by the staging tests (see Chapter 6). If a small tumour that has not spread is found, then an operation, radiotherapy, or chemotherapy will be used to try to cure the patient. When more extensive tumour that cannot be cured is discovered, decisions regarding treatment must weigh the potential benefits against the possible side-effects of the treatment. However, although intensive treatment with the aim of cure is not advisable in these circumstances, treatment will not be abandoned—the goals are changed to containing the disease and its symptoms.

Patients and their families usually need time to discuss what has been found by the various staging tests with their doctor who may, in the past, have been reluctant to discuss the diagnosis of cancer and what it means to the patient (see Chapter 12). Indeed, doctors often cover what are their own inadequacies by rationalizing that the patient 'cannot take it' or they 'would not understand'. The truth is most people are far tougher than they themselves or their doctor appreciates. Although rules cannot be made, it is usually helpful for everyone concerned if there is an honest and open discussion of the problem. This should be as optimistic as the situation allows but also needs to be realistic.

Hopefully this book will answer some of the questions that arise, but it is most important to try to develop a close, understanding relationship with doctors and nurses. Books like this can be a useful prop, but nothing can replace the support and care that family, friends, doctors, and nurses can give.

Because no attempt has been made to conceal the truth, parts of this book may make depressing reading. These sections were included because I considered that anyone reading this book will want the undistorted facts.

7
Treatment of non-small-cell cancer

This chapter is concerned with the treatment of the three types of lung cancer (squamous, adenocarcinoma, and large-cell carcinoma) that are commonly lumped together as non-small-cell lung cancer (see p. 6). They are grouped together because they seem to behave in a similar fashion and because an operation to remove the cancer gives the best chance for cure in all three. Although operations to remove a part of the lung had been attempted earlier, the first successful operation to remove a cancerous lung was done in 1933. The patient, a 48-year-old doctor, recovered well from the operation and continued to work for many years. Nowadays operations to remove part or all of a lung are routine and only carry a small risk. Improvements in the operation have come from new surgical techniques and, more importantly, better anaesthesia and post-operative care. Although removal of the cancer can be curative, this is only likely when the tumour is small and has not spread outside the lung.

SURGERY

SELECTION OF PATIENTS FOR AN OPERATION

Because surgery is often the best or only chance of cure it is important that patients are not denied the possibility of an operation unless there is unquestionable evidence that an operation would not be useful. Selection is therefore designed to pick out those patients who will definitely *not* benefit from surgery and in whom an unnecessary operation can be avoided. The tests used to select patients are discussed briefly in Chapter 6.

Once the diagnosis of non-small-cell lung cancer has been made patients will be checked to see if their tumour can be removed. The first step is simply to consider, based on the chest X-ray and appearance on looking down into the lungs (bronchoscopy; see p. 35), whether the cancer is small enough to operate on. If it is, the patient will be examined for signs of disease outside the chest and appropriate tests will be done. Staging tests (see Chapter 6) may be used to look for tumour in the liver,

50 Lung cancer: the facts

bones and possibly the bone marrow. If these tests are all normal, and the cancer seems to only involve the lung, the surgeon may organize further tests to see how widespread it is within the chest. These include assessment of the size and position of the tumour using mediastinoscopy or mediastinotomy (see p. 41), and/or CT scanning (see p. 40). The major findings that would suggest that an operation is not going to be useful are:

- Cancer that has spread outside the chest or to the other lung.
- Cancer invading or pressing on the major airways near their main division in the chest (the carina; see Fig. 8, p. 31).
- Cancer invading the trachea (the main airway into the chest; see Fig. 8, p. 31).
- Invasion of the major blood vessels or heart. Involvement of lymph nodes in the centre of the chest (mediastinum) or on the other side of the chest.
- Involvement of lymph nodes at the root of the neck.
- Fluid around the lungs (pleural effusion; see p. 85).
- Loss of voice and hoarseness caused by pressure on one of the nerves to the vocal chords (see p. 91).

Lung function tests

If none of these features are found, an operation may be beneficial but, before it can be planned, tests to see how good lung function is are carried out. Because one lung may need to be removed it is important to see if the other lung is working well enough to be able to cope after the operation. As well as measuring simple exercise tolerance there are sophisticated ways of measuring the lungs' capacity for breathing, all of which are simple and painless. Some patients will have a series of tests called 'lung function studies'. During these, they are asked to breathe both normally and as hard as they can into various machines. If there is doubt about the ability of the other lung to work sufficiently well by itself, special tests measuring only the function of that lung can be done in a few hospitals. At the time lung function is being assessed, general health and fitness to stand the operation and anaesthetic will be judged.

This whole process of selecting patients for operation sounds complicated, although in most cases the process is quite simple. Figure 11, a flow diagram, summarizes the process and types of tests used.

Treatment of non-small-cell cancer

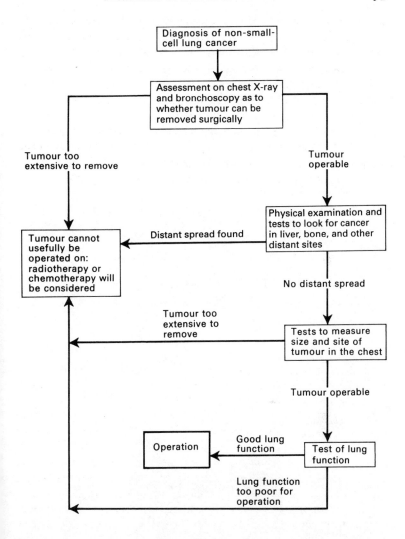

Fig. 11 Flow diagram showing how patients with non-small-cell lung cancer are selected for an operation.

OPERATIONS FOR NON-SMALL-CELL LUNG CANCER

After this rigorous selection procedure it seems likely that between one-quarter and one-third of all patients might benefit from an operation. The pie diagram in Figure 12(a) shows the proportion of patients selected for an exploratory operation (a thoracotomy) and the percentage who underwent actual removal of part or all of a lung (resection). These data, based on the experience of one hospital treating nearly 2000 patients over nearly 20 years, show that a little less than one-quarter of patients are able to have an operation to remove their tumour. The proportion of patients who are found to have disease that is too extensive to remove when their chest is opened up will, of course, depend on how intensive the initial staging tests were (see p. 40). These days most hospitals should expect less than 10 per cent of the patients they operate on to have a tumour that is too extensive to be removed (Fig. 12(b)).

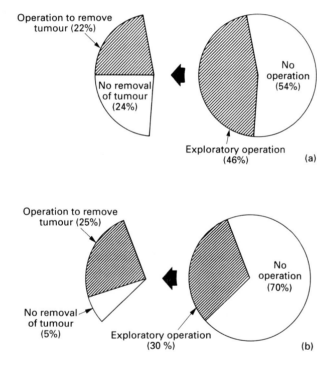

Fig. 12 The percentage of patients who undergo an operation for removal of non-small-cell lung cancer. (a) The experience of one hospital in the 1960s and 1970s; (b) current pattern of surgical care.

Treatment of non-small-cell cancer

The type of operation that is done will depend on the size of the tumour, its position, and the general health of the patient—in particular the condition of their heart and other lung. The actual extent of the operation must be decided on by the surgeon once they have opened the chest and can weigh-up the situation. The aim of the operation is to remove all known disease whilst conserving as much normal lung as possible.

Such a conservative approach, when feasible, is just as good as a more extensive operation, although removal of the whole lung and its lymph nodes (a total pneumonectomy) always used to be done, even when the tumour was very small. This type of operation obviously carries greater risks than removal of just part of a lung.

Lung operations can be carried out with the patient either face-up or face-down using an incision over the front or back of the chest. It is far more common, however, to place the patient on their side with the tumour uppermost. The chest is opened using an incision that usually starts just below the nipple in front and curves backwards just below the tip of the shoulder blade almost to the spine (Fig. 13). The various layers

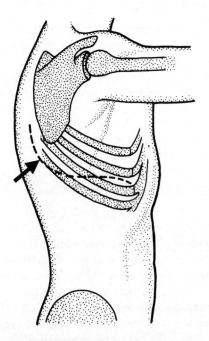

Fig. 13 The usual incision for a thoracotomy.

54   Lung cancer: the facts

of muscle below the skin are divided and the inside of the chest is opened either by removing part of a rib or cutting through the muscles between two ribs. This operation to explore the chest is called a thoracotomy; the surgeon, having opened the chest, is then in a position to examine the lung and its lymph nodes. If necessary small pieces of tissue can be examined on the spot, the tissue is frozen solid before being cut into thin sections for microscopic examination (a frozen section).

The surgeon will at this point decide if an operation is going to be possible and, if it is, how extensive it will need to be. The usual operations are removal of the whole lung (pneumonectomy), removal of part of the lung supplied by a main airway (lobectomy), or removal of a part or wedge of lung (segmentectomy). More extensive operations to remove the lung and adjacent ribs or the lining (pleura) over the lungs may be done in special cases. Smaller operations, called sleeve resections, to conserve as much normal lung as possible when the patient has poor lung function are another option.

AFTER THE OPERATION

The operation is done under general anaesthetic. Patients are given an injection in the ward (a premedication) before being taken to the operating room, and often feel drowsy and remember little until they awake in the recovery room after the operation. Frequently patients are not even aware that they have had the operation when they wake up. Most hospitals keep patients in a special intensive care unit for a day or two after this type of operation. This is because there are specially trained nursing staff and doctors to keep a close eye on the patient's condition after what is a fairly major operation.

Patients will be monitored carefully for the first few days after their operation and several special techniques are used to help them get over it more quickly:

- A drain is left in the chest to help remove air from around the lung. This tube is connected to a bottle containing water. This prevents air getting back into the space around the lung while allowing air to escape from the chest when the patient coughs and raises the pressure in their chest. If necessary, this bottle can be connected to a pump that helps suck the air from the chest.
- Most patients will be given oxygen, usually by a tube under the nose, after the operation. Some patients who have difficulty breathing will

Treatment of non-small-cell cancer

be sedated and have a tube left in their main airway to help with their breathing using a mechanical ventilator. Once the lungs are working well enough this tube, which is similar to that used during the operation, can be removed.

- Physiotherapy will be started shortly after the operation because it is important to clear secretions from the lungs. Because it is uncomfortable to cough after the operation, patients need encouragement and advice on how to reduce the pain. Coughing is made less painful if support is given over the ribs next to the scar. Patients will be asked to move their legs around in bed and will get out of bed (for short periods) within a day or so of surgery. It is important to keep active to reduce the risk of clots developing in the veins in the legs.
- Frequent checks of pulse, blood pressure, and breathing will be made in the first hours after the operation and blood will be taken from an artery in the side of the wrist to check oxygen levels in the blood.
- When the lung has fully re-expanded (if only part was removed) the chest tubes will be removed. The length of time the tube is left in the chest varies from patient to patient and may be anywhere from three to seven or more days after the operation. The adhesive tape holding the tube is removed and the tube quickly pulled out with the patient breathing out. A pressure dressing is put on the wound and another chest X-ray will be done to make sure that the lung remains expanded.
- The sutures (stitches) are removed about a week after the operation.
- There is no getting over the fact that operations on the chest cause a lot of pain and discomfort and large doses of pain-killers will be needed for some days after the operation.

REHABILITATION

Within a few days most patients are up and about and gradually increasing the amount of exercise that they take. Many are ready for discharge 10–14 days after the operation, although they may benefit from a period of convalescence. The wound will be painful during the first few days after surgery but this will gradually lessen and can be reduced by pain-killing injections and, later, by tablets. However, some patients will have discomfort and altered feeling around the scar for quite some time. The need for any additional anti-cancer treatment will depend on the findings at operation but radiotherapy (see p. 58) and/or chemotherapy (see p.61) may be recommended.

56 Lung cancer: the facts

POSSIBLE COMPLICATIONS OF SURGERY

Unfortunately, all treatments have risks attached to them. Despite careful selection of patients for surgery on the lungs, a very small proportion die soon after what is a major operation; this is usually due to heart problems in older patients. However, the vast majority of patients recover from surgery. The important potential complications of surgery on the lung include:

- Excessive bleeding during the operation—this is rarely difficult to control if patients are selected carefully.
- Changes in heart rhythm (cardiac dysrhythmias) or heart attacks. Most dysrhythmias cause no symptoms and can be controlled with drugs.
- Persistent leakage of air into the chest requiring prolonged drainage. Very occasionally another operation is needed to seal an air leak from the main airway which was 'tied off' during the operation.
- Collapse or infection in the other lung. This will require physiotherapy and antibiotics.
- Infection in the chest between the lung and chest wall (an empyema). This requires drainage of pus by a tube through the chest, as well as antibiotics.
- Formation of clots in the veins in the legs (deep venous thrombosis—DVT), which can result in a clot breaking off and going to the lungs (a pulmonary embolus). Drugs to 'thin' the blood and prevent clot formation (heparin and warfarin) may be needed if a clot does develop.

However, most patients will have few problems and will be able to leave hospital within a short period.

RESULTS OF SURGERY

These depend to a large extent on selecting the right patients. If staging is done meticulously then all the patients likely to benefit will have an operation and unnecessary surgery will be avoided in those who cannot be helped. However, despite removal of all or part of a lung, only about one-third of patients undergoing such an operation are cured. The extent of disease (TNM system; see p. 39) is used to divide patients up into three groups. The chance of cure is best for those with the least disease and becomes worse when it is more extensive (Table 9): unfortunately

Treatment of non-small-cell cancer   57

most patients present with extensive disease. If the chances of cure by surgery are looked at according to the type of non-small-cell cancer (see p. 6), it seems that those with squamous cancer do a little better (about 35 per cent surviving for 5 years) than those with large-cell anaplastic or adenocarcinoma (about 25 per cent surviving for 5 years).

Table 9. Survival after surgery for non-small-cell cancer

Extent of disease at operation (TNM stage)	Percentage of patients surviving for 5 or more years
Stage I	53
Stage II	29
Stage III	16

It is difficult to say when a patient can be regarded as 'cured' but most patients whose disease is going to grow back develop new symptoms (relapse) within 2 years. The chances of cure increase the longer a patient goes without recurrent disease, and relapses after 4 or 5 years are rare.

Because patients who have had an operation to remove their tumour are at risk of the cancer growing back, doctors have tried using radiotherapy or drug therapy immediately after an operation (see p. 49) to try to prevent this. This approach, called adjuvant therapy, is discussed on page 63.

TREATMENT WHEN AN OPERATION CANNOT BE DONE

Unfortunately the majority of patients (65–75 per cent) cannot have an operation to remove their cancer as the tumour is too extensive locally or has spread outside the chest. In addition to these patients, 10 or more per cent of those who have an operation are found to have a tumour that cannot be removed (see p. 52). There are also some patients with a small operable tumour who are too unwell or whose lungs do not work well enough to allow an operation. The treatment for such inoperable

58 Lung cancer: the facts

tumours will be chosen for the individual patients and may include radiotherapy and drug treatment (chemotherapy) as well as treatment aimed at helping reduce specific symptoms.

RADIOTHERAPY

Radiotherapy is the use of X-rays and other types of so-called ionizing radiation to treat cancer. High doses of radiation damage cells and can often kill them, especially if they are dividing. Cancers are often more sensitive to the effects of ionizing radiation than surrounding tissues— probably because they repair the damage less well than normal cells. Unfortunately the dose of radiation that can be given is limited by the amount of damage done to normal tissues, and because of this it is often not possible to give enough treatment to kill all the cancer cells. More details on the way radiotherapy works are given in the books on cancer treatments listed on page 118.

The first visit to a radiotherapy department is spent checking the patient's general health, stage of the tumour, and then planning how the treatment is to be given. More X-rays will probably be taken to outline the extent of the cancer and an individual programme of treatment designed. The area to be treated is drawn out in a purple dye on the patient's skin. This is to make sure that treatment is given to the correct area each time and the patient will be warned not to wash it off. Alternatively, small tattoos (dots only) are used to mark the corners of the radiotherapy 'field'. This stage of planning treatment may take up to several hours, although treatment itself only takes a few minutes.

Because it is safer and more effective to divide the treatment up, radiotherapy is usually given four or five times a week; each treatment being called a 'fraction'. Some treatment courses take around three to four weeks to complete. Treatment is given with large and rather daunting machines, and it is important to remember that all the careful measurement and complicated machinery is designed to give a very precisely measured dose of radiation treatment in a safe manner. When treatment is being given patients are left alone in the room, although the radiographer can see them through a special window or on a television screen and can talk to them through an intercom system. Each treatment will only take a few minutes. Sometimes radiotherapy treatment is given in a single dose or a very short course rather than over several weeks.

Treatment of non-small-cell cancer 59

Side-effects of radiotherapy

It is inevitable that radiation will cause some side-effects, as the treatment will always include normal tissues around the cancer. The type of side-effect will, of course, depend largely on the part of the body being treated. In lung cancer the areas that are commonly treated include the chest, bones, and sometimes the brain. Common side-effects include:

- *Cough.* Inflammation of the lung caused by the radiotherapy will often lead to a dry, irritating cough that can be troublesome; it can be treated with a cough suppressant and, if severe, with corticosteroids (see p. 92).
- *Pain on swallowing.* The oesophagus (gullet) is sensitive to radiation and radiotherapy treatment to the centre of the chest will often cause temporary pain and discomfort on eating or swallowing. This comes on towards the end of the course of radiotherapy and will gradually subside once treatment has been discontinued. If it is troublesome tell your radiotherapist. Mucaine—a local anaesthetic mixture—can be used before meals and drinking to reduce the discomfort on swallowing.
- *Tiredness.* This is very common during radiation treatment and may build up during the course of the treatment. It will usually improve fairly quickly in the first few weeks after stopping treatment.
- *Nausea and loss of appetite.* As well as tiredness, some patients will notice nausea if large areas of the body are being treated with radiotherapy. In lung cancer it is not usually a great problem and those suffering from it can be helped by anti-sickness medicines.
- *Sleepiness and loss of concentration and memory.* Starting about 6 weeks after treatment, sleepiness and loss of concentration and memory may affect some patients who have radiation to their brain. This returns to normal after a month or two, only affecting a minority of patients.
- *Reddening and soreness of the skin.* This is not a problem with radiotherapy for lung cancer, although patients will be advised to care for the skin being treated by avoiding putting perfumes, soap, cosmetics, hot water bottles, UV or heat lamps on the area. Ointments should not be used on the area without first consulting your radiotherapist.

The side-effects of radiotherapy can be made worse when some anti-cancer drugs (chemotherapy) are given at the same time; use of irradiation and chemotherapy must therefore be planned carefully.

60 Lung cancer: the facts

Before starting any treatment with radiotherapy it is important to find out as much as possible about the treatment and its side-effects. Some of the queries will have been answered in this section but it is important to ask about your own treatment, as every radiotherapy treatment plan is individualized. Table 10 suggests some possible questions.

Table 10. Suggested questions to ask about radiotherapy

Why do I need radiotherapy?
Are there any alternative treatments?
Which part of my body will be treated?
How often is the treatment given and how long does each treatment take?
How long will it take to complete the course of treatment?
Can I drive home after treatment or will I need transport?
Will I feel tired?
Will I feel sick?
Does the treatment cause soreness on swallowing?
Are there any other side-effects during treatment?
Are there any side-effects that may appear after treatment?
Should I take any special precautions during treatment?

What can be achieved with radiotherapy?

This will, of course, depend very much on the size of the cancer and whether it has spread. The best results are seen in those patients who have a small tumour that could have been surgically removed if they had been fit enough to withstand the operation (see p. 51). In this un-common situation, high doses of radiotherapy are given in an attempt to cure the patient. Various treatment schedules have been used but treatment is usually given to quite high doses (55–65 Grays; a Gray being the measurement of the dose of radiation used). Similarly, patients with small tumours that cannot be removed surgically may be treated with high doses of radiation. When radiotherapy is used in this way to try to cure patients with small tumours the results are not as good as those achieved with surgery; up to one in ten patients survives for more than five years. However, the great majority of the rest benefit by shrinkage of their tumour and control of symptoms. Clearly the side-effects of radio-therapy (see p. 59) are more pronounced when high doses are used to try to eradicate the cancer.

Treatment of non-small-cell cancer 61

Much more common is the situation where a patient has an extensive tumour in the chest that cannot be removed surgically or there is spread of the cancer outside the chest. In these situations the aims of radiotherapy are altered: it is given to try to reduce unpleasant symptoms and, if possible, to prolong life. Cure is, unfortunately, not an achievable goal for these patients, and care must therefore be taken in selecting treatment. It is essential that there is a significant benefit from treatment, which outweighs the side-effects. Because of this, many radiotherapists will only give radiation therapy if the patient is troubled by symptoms, whilst others may use radiation to try to prevent symptoms developing. There is little information to say which approach is best but many British radiotherapists withhold treatment until symptoms occur. The symptoms that can be helped by radiotherapy include:

- coughing up blood;
- breathlessness caused by collapse of part of a lung;
- swelling of the neck or face caused by pressure on large veins in the chest (superior vena caval obstruction; see Fig. 17, p. 84);
- pain caused by tumour in a bone;
- symptoms caused by tumour in the brain or tumour pressing on a nerve.

Although radiotherapy is often very effective at shrinking the tumour and reducing these types of symptoms, there is unfortunately little evidence that it causes greatly prolonged life. Because of this the dose of radiotherapy used is usually smaller (30–50 Grays), so that there are fewer side-effects. Failure of radiotherapy to cure patients with extensive tumours probably reflects the fact that the tumour had already spread to other parts of the body before treatment, as well as the relative lack of sensitivity of non-small-cell lung cancer to radiotherapy.

DRUG THERAPY FOR NON-SMALL-CELL LUNG CANCER

The treatment of this type of lung cancer with drugs (chemotherapy) has been slow to develop because of a lack of really effective drugs. While combinations of drugs can be used to cure some cancers, even when they are in an advanced state, only a minority of patients with lung cancer are at all responsive to drug treatment.

All anti-cancer drugs cause side-effects, some of which may be severe. It is, therefore, of great importance that the potential benefits of treatment (tumour shrinkage and control of symptoms) are carefully weighed

62 **Lung cancer: the facts**

against the known disadvantages. Currently it is not possible to cure non-small-cell lung cancer with drugs and the aim of any treatment must be to relieve symptoms and, if possible, prolong life with a minimum of side-effects.

A number of anti-cancer drugs, when used on their own, can shrink tumours by at least half in some patients (Table 11). As can be seen from the table, only about one-quarter of patients have a good response to treatment with a single drug and in most cases this only lasts a few months. So, although single-drug chemotherapy does cause tumour shrinkage (called a remission or response) for some patients, it rarely prolongs life and, because of this, several drugs may be used together in combinations.

Table 11. Response rate for single drugs in the chemotherapy of non-small-cell lung cancer

Drug	Proportion of patients responding* (%)
Vindesine	23
Mitomycin C	27
Cisplatin	25
Ifosfamide	20
Adriamycin	18
Etopopside	15

* An objective response is regarded as a shrinkage of the tumour volume by one-half or greater that lasts for more than 1 month.

Combination chemotherapy

In nearly all cancers where drug treatment is curative a combination of drugs is needed to give the best chance of response and cure. Several recent combinations of drugs (Table 12) have been shown to cause measurable shrinkage of tumour in a good proportion of patients with non-small-cell lung cancer. However, many of these responses are still short-lived and as such treatments have a lot of side-effects it is most important to see if combinations of drugs will improve the *quality* as well as the *length* of life for patients with advanced lung cancer.

Treatment of non-small-cell cancer 63

Table 12. Response rate for selected combinations of drugs in the chemotherapy of non-small-cell lung cancer

Drugs	Percentage of patients responding [*]
Vindesine + cisplatin	43
Etoposide + cisplatin	43
Mitomycin C + vinblastine + cisplatin	53
5-fluorouracil + vincristine + mitomycin C	36
Mitomycin C + ifosfamide + cisplatin	63

[*] An objective response is regarded as a shrinkage of the tumour volume by one-half or greater that lasts for more than 1 month.

A suggested list of questions to ask about chemotherapy is shown in Table 13 and detailed information on the side-effects of chemotherapy can be found by reading the books on cancer therapy listed on page 118.

Table 13. Suggested questions to ask about chemotherapy

Why is drug treatment needed?
What are the aims of chemotherapy?
What drugs will be used and how are they given?
Are there any immediate or long-term side-effects?
Do I need to come into hospital for treatment?
How often is treatment given?
How long will the treatment go on for?
What are the chances that it will benefit me?
Is the treatment part of a trial?

Until we are able to show that chemotherapy benefits patients with lung cancer, routine use of drugs cannot be recommended. After an attempt has been made to cure a patient with surgery or radiotherapy, chemotherapy is currently being considered as a way of improving chances of survival (so-called adjuvant chemotherapy). Although drugs have been used in this way, such trials remain highly speculative and this approach is not yet regarded as a standard way of treating patients.

In the past 10 years chemotherapy for non-small-cell lung cancer has made some small advances but until we can build on these it seems unlikely that many patients will have real benefit from its use.

COMBINED THERAPY OF NON-SMALL-CELL LUNG CANCER

In patients who have had, or who are about to undergo, surgical removal of a lung tumour, radiation and/or chemotherapy may be used to try to improve the results of the operation. The idea of the additional treatment is to reduce the size of the tumour if radiotherapy is given before an operation, or to try and ensure that all the tumour in the chest is eradicated if radiotherapy is used after surgery. Chemotherapy is given with the intention of treating the tumour in the lung and any cancer that may have already spread outside the chest.

Radiotherapy

Radiotherapy followed by surgery is sometimes the best treatment for patients with cancers confined high up in the apex of the lung (so-called superior sulcus tumours; Fig. 14).

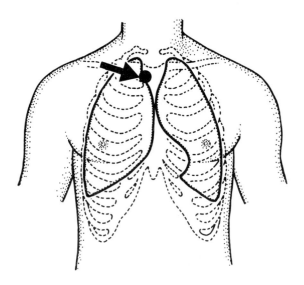

Fig. 14 The area in the lungs (arrow) where a superior sulcus tumour develops. This may be on either side of the chest.

Treatment of non-small-cell cancer   65

Tumours in this part of the lung are liable to involve the complex of nerves coming out from the neck to supply the arm. They may also invade bones in the upper chest and neck and are therefore liable to cause pain and weakness in the arm. Radiotherapy, sometimes together with surgery, can give good control of this type of lung cancer. Because these tumours seem to grow more slowly and to spread later than similar tumours in other parts of the lung, extensive operations to remove them are more often successful. Some hospitals will use radiotherapy in selected patients (usually in a low dose—30 Grays given over a couple of weeks) followed, if possible, by surgical removal of the tumour about a month later.

Chemotherapy

Until recently, there has been no evidence that drug therapy (chemotherapy) used together with surgery increases the chances of cure. Indeed, in some cases it can be harmful—13 clinical trials including 5333 patients failed to show any improvement in survival, and all reported side-effects from chemotherapy. However, a recent trial comparing chemotherapy and radiotherapy together with radiotherapy alone seem to show a definite advantage for the combined treatment and this trend is being followed up.

IMMUNOTHERAPY

This is the attempt to control or cure cancer by manipulating the body's immune system. There was much interest in immunotherapy in the 1970s but its failure to produce any useful benefit in most patients has meant that it is now less commonly used. The techniques used were crude and non-specific and, looking back, it is not surprising that they failed to help patients. More recently, increasingly sophisticated methods of using the immune system are being developed, although they remain experimental and of unproven value.

It was originally noticed that patients who developed a postoperative infection in the space between the lung and chest wall (an empyema; see p. 85) seemed to have a better chance of cure than those who had an uncomplicated operation. Because of this, surgeons in New York treated a group of patients having an operation by instilling BCG (the preparation used to immunize against tuberculosis) into the pleural space to cause an emphysema, which they hoped would stimulate the body's im-

66 Lung cancer: the facts

mune system. They found that those patients with the smallest amount of disease appeared to survive longer if they had the BCG treatment. However, despite excitement at this discovery, further trials of this treatment have failed to show any benefit.

Other trials using BCG and another drug called levamisole, which is said to stimulate the immune system, have also failed to benefit patients. More recently drugs such as interferon and interleukin-2 have been tested. These are naturally occurring substances normally produced by the body in response to infection and can be given in high doses. So far, despite marked side-effects, they have failed to be useful in lung cancer, although they are active in some other cancers.

THE OUTLOOK FOR THE FUTURE

Surgery has reached a plateau and further improvements in techniques are unlikely to cure more patients because the major problem is one of spread of the cancer outside the lung before the diagnosis can be made. However, continued improvement in our ability to detect and measure cancer inside or outside the chest will reduce the need for unnecessary operations because we will be able to recognize a much greater proportion of patients who have a tumour that is too advanced to be successfully removed.

Radiotherapy suffers from the same problem as surgery; it is a local treatment that does not affect cancer cells that have spread outside the area being treated. Cancer cells that are short of oxygen are more resistant to radiotherapy and, because of this, drugs called radiosensitizers are being tested. Many cells in tumours have a poor blood supply and are therefore short of oxygen. Radiosensitizers have an effect equivalent to increasing the oxygen level in the cancer and make the tumour cells that are short of oxygen more sensitive to radiation damage. Their use remains experimental, although it is clear that they are unlikely to result in many more cures because the main problem in lung cancer is the tumour (often unrecognized) that has spread outside the chest.

Drug treatments that will get to cancer cells wherever they may be in the body are obviously of paramount importance but remain an unfulfilled but an exciting prospect for the future.

8
Treatment of small-cell lung cancer

In contrast to the other common lung cancers (see p. 6), the best chance for cure in this disease does not lie with surgery. This is because, in nearly all cases, the tumour has spread widely in the chest and to other parts of the body by the time of diagnosis. Fortunately small-cell lung cancer is much more responsive to treatment with drugs and radiation, and these treatments are now the mainstay of therapy.

As it is not so important to decide who may benefit from surgery, staging for small-cell lung cancer is very simple—dividing patients into those with disease confined to one side of the chest and those with more extensive disease (see Table 5, p. 38). Patients with localized disease, not surprisingly, more often respond to treatment and live longer than those with extensive disease.

TREATMENT

CHEMOTHERAPY

When single anti-cancer drugs are used in this disease about 40 per cent of patients have a useful response to treatment. This effect is produced by a number of different types of anti-cancer drugs (Table 14). More importantly, not only do single anti-cancer drugs shrink the tumour, they also increase survival. Randomized studies 20 years ago showed that one anti-cancer drug (cyclophosphamide) improved the survival of patients with widespread small-cell lung cancer compared with the survival of patients not receiving chemotherapy. However, when used singly drugs rarely cause complete disappearance of tumour, and it has become common practice to use several anti-cancer drugs together in a combination to get the best effect.

In nearly all cancers sensitive to chemotherapy, combinations of two or more drugs are much more effective at shrinking tumours, and hopefully at curing patients. When several anti-cancer drugs are used together the number of patients responding increases dramatically (Table 15) and many more have complete disappearance of all their detectable disease (a

Lung cancer: the facts

Table 14. Response rate for single anti-cancer drugs used alone in small-cell cancer

Drug	Response rate (%)*
Cyclophosphamide	38
Ifosfamide	63
Nitrogen mustard	44
Vincristine	42
Etoposide	40
Adriamycin	30
Methotrexate	30
Procarbazine	47
Cisplatin	23

* Response is defined as a shrinkage of the tumour volume by at least one-half that lasts for at least 1 month.

complete remission). It has now become customary to use combinations of three or four drugs, and many such combinations are available from the 30 or so anti-cancer drugs in current use.

Table 15. Response rates for combination chemotherapy in small-cell lung cancer

Stage and number of drugs in combination	Response rate (%)*	Complete response rate (%) †
Localized disease ‡		
Three drugs	88	44
Four or more drugs	89	54
Extensive disease §		
Two drugs	46	21
Three drugs	50	27
Four or more drugs	48	30

* Defined as shrinkage or the tumour volume by at least 50% lasting for more than 1 month.
† Defined as complete disappearance of all evidence of the tumour for at least 1 month.
‡ Tumour confined to one side of the chest only.
§ Tumour which is more widespread than one side of the chest.

Treatment of small-cell lung cancer 69

Most combinations include drugs given by injection into a vein, with or without tablets, once every three weeks. All anti-cancer drugs cause some side-effects, and more specific details about chemotherapy can be found in books included in the booklist (see p. 118). It is important, however, to ask about any chemotherapy you may receive and Table 13 (p. 63) suggests some possible questions.

Although it is beyond the scope of this book to detail the side-effects of the many drug combinations used in this disease, some of the common ones include:

- tiredness, lethargy, and loss of appetite during treatment;
- hair loss (especially with adriamycin, etoposide, cyclophosphamide, and ifosfamide—the hair always grows back afterwards);
- anaemia;
- susceptibility to infection because of a low white cell count (the infection fighting cells in the blood);
- tendency towards bruising or bleeding because of a low platelet count (the clotting cells in the blood);
- pins and needles in the hands and feet with some drugs. This is usually temporary but you should tell your doctor if it occurs as the treatment may need to be adjusted.

It is important to remember that not everyone will have all of these side-effects, and it is essential that you discuss your treatment fully before it starts.

RADIOTHERAPY

The results of radiation, when used as the main treatment for small-cell lung cancer, have proved to be similar to surgery, as radiation is essentially a localized treatment and we know that spread of the tumour occurs at an early stage in nearly all patients. However, when patients are treated with chemotherapy alone the tumour sometimes grows back in the chest, despite a good response to the drug treatment. Trials to test radiotherapy given after initial treatment with drugs have shown that there is a modest increase in survival when both treatments are used in localized disease. Because of the side-effects of the two treatments together, some hospitals do not routinely use this approach whilst others do. When there is 'extensive' disease there is no evidence that radiotherapy improves the results of chemotherapy alone.

70 Lung cancer: the facts

The best way to combine radiotherapy with chemotherapy is not known, although when both are used at the same time there are undoubtedly many more side-effects. When radiation therapy is used it is given in much the same way as that given for non-small-cell lung cancer (see p. 58).

SURGERY

In those patients who have a solitary tumour of small-cell cancer in the periphery of their lung, without any evidence of spread, there is about a one in three chance of cure with surgery. Unfortunately very few patients with this disease have such a small amount of tumour, and in general surgery cannot be used because this cancer spreads at an early stage.

Despite combining radiotherapy and chemotherapy, many patients who have a complete response still have the tumour grow back in the lung. Because of this, some hospitals are exploring whether surgery, to remove part or all of the lung, is useful soon after patients have had a good response to chemotherapy. This type of treatment is very new and no conclusions about its efficacy can yet be drawn.

If surgery is used, then the techniques are similar to those employed for non-small-cell lung cancer (see p. 51).

IMMUNOTHERAPY

Various attempts to stimulate the body's immune system to overcome the cancer have been made. There was a lot of interest in this area in the 1970s but the results have been disappointing and nearly all randomized trials (see p. 65) have shown that treatment with BCG, *Corynebacterium parvum* (an infectious organism), and levamisole have not improved the patient's chances of survival.

All these techniques are rather crude and non-specific, and scientists are continuing to try to develop new and more specific methods of using the body's immune system to destroy cancer cells. However, these remain experimental, and immunotherapy is best avoided unless it is in part of a trial. The newly developed drugs interferon and interleukin-2 (see p. 66) are not useful in this disease and cause a lot of side-effects.

SPREAD TO THE BRAIN

Because small-cell lung cancer grows and spreads rapidly there is a tendency for the central nervous system (brain and spinal cord) to

Treatment of small-cell lung cancer 71

become involved. Unfortunately drugs do not enter the brain and spinal cord very well and, despite drug treatment, there is a tendency for patients to develop tumours in the brain even if they had a good response to chemotherapy.

Because of this, patients who have responded to chemotherapy treatment are often given radiotherapy to the brain in an attempt to make sure that the tumour does not develop in the brain. Such radiotherapy is usually given over about 2–3 weeks and is usually not upsetting, although temporary sleepiness and loss of memory and concentration may occur about 6–8 weeks later in some patients. Numerous trials have tested the effectiveness of such prophylactic brain irradiation and there is no doubt that this treatment reduces the risk of developing of symptoms from tumour in the brain. It will, however, also cause hair loss or delay hair regrowth in people who have already lost their hair during chemotherapy. There has been concern, particularly in the United States where higher doses of radiation have been used, that such a pattern of treatment may sometimes affect brain tissues in those who survive more than a few years after treatment. These possible complications are being studied at present and there is greater caution in use of high doses of irradiation.

CURRENT RECOMMENDATIONS FOR TREATMENT

Despite improvements in treatment over the past ten years there are still many unanswered questions and there is a need for new and more effective therapies. However, some recommendations can be made.

LOCALIZED DISEASE

- When the tumour is small, in the outer part of the lung, and there is no sign of spread on careful staging, an operation to remove the tumour is indicated. This should probably be followed with chemotherapy for about 6 months.
- When there is more extensive local tumour, combination chemotherapy is used and will get rid of all visible disease in more than half the patients.
- Many hospitals give radiotherapy to the site of the tumour when the patient has completed an initial period of chemotherapy.
- Once a complete response has been gained some hospitals will stop treatment, but others will give further chemotherapy. Whilst the

72 Lung cancer: the facts

need for this 'maintenance' treatment is debatable, it seems likely that prolonged treatment is *not* very useful.

- Patients achieving a good response should be considered for prophylactic brain radiotherapy.
- Most patients with localized disease show a good response but some will unfortunately relapse, although up to 15–20 per cent may survive for long periods without the tumour recurring and are cured.
- Patients relapsing from a good response may benefit from more chemotherapy, but those failing to respond to the first treatment rarely do well with more drug therapy.

EXTENSIVE DISEASE

- Combination chemotherapy should always be used as the initial treatment, although even this may not be helpful in sick patients with very extensive small-cell lung cancer.
- There is no role for surgery or routine radiotherapy to the chest.
- Patients showing a very good response to treatment may be considered for prophylactic brain irradiation.
- Unfortunately less than one-quarter of patients have a complete response and very few are potentially curable.
- More chemotherapy is indicated for those who relapse after a good response, although it may be best avoided in patients who are very unwell because of their tumour.
- Patients failing to respond to initial chemotherapy do not usually benefit from more drug treatment.

THE OUTLOOK IN SMALL-CELL LUNG CANCER

The development and increasing use of combination chemotherapy has greatly improved the results of treatment for this type of lung cancer. Because it is such a rapidly growing disease, many patients in the past died within a few weeks or months of diagnosis, despite surgery or radiotherapy. This was because the tumour had already spread widely throughout the body before diagnosis.

Drug treatment is able to cause tumour regression in a great majority of patients and complete disappearance of all disease in a good proportion. Although long-term disease control or 'cure' is only likely in some patients with localized disease, the majority of patients with small-cell

Treatment of small-cell lung cancer 73

lung cancer benefit from treatment despite the side-effects. Many patients are able to go back to work and to lead a useful life and most will have a prolongation of their life for a year or more, even if cure is not possible.

Of all the various types of lung cancer, small-cell has undergone the greatest change in treatment and results. It is likely that the improvement in chemotherapy will continue and may include other types of treatment (surgery, radiotherapy, immunotherapy, etc.). Survival in small-cell lung cancer is much better than it was 10 years ago and there is no reason to believe that the next 10 years will not show a similar improvement. New drugs (see p. 109) are constantly being looked for and new techniques such as hyperthermia (see p. 80) and phototherapy (see p. 78) are being developed. Recent discoveries of growth factors (see Chapter 15) that can stimulate the bone marrow to produce more white cells (infection-fighting cells) may mean that more intensive drug treatment may be possible and bone marrow transplantation (using the patient's own marrow to protect them from the side-effects of very-high-dose chemotherapy) is already being tested.

9

Treatment of other lung tumours

MESOTHELIOMAS

Although tumours of the lining of the lung (the pleura) were first described as long as two centuries ago, there has been debate until recently whether it is a separate tumour. The increasing incidence of these mesotheliomas, understanding of their biology and their clear-cut relationship to asbestos exposure have, however, become clear in the past 20 years.

The pleura (see p. 31) is the lining that wraps itself around the lung and covers the inside of the chest wall. The space between the two layers of the pleura is the pleural cavity; the two layers are normally in contact, with a small amount of fluid between them to provide lubrication. The whole of the abdominal cavity and its contents is covered with a similar lining (peritoneum) and mesotheliomas of the peritoneum also occur, although they are less common.

Studies into the cause of mesothelioma have shown that up to 80 per cent of all cases develop in individuals clearly exposed to asbestos dust. Exposure may be at work (see Table 3, p. 13) or in the home or local environment. Often there is a long delay between exposure to asbestos and the eventual development of a mesothelioma. This interval, known as the latent period, ranges from 10 to 65 years, but is usually 20–40 years. The exposure may be very brief; unlike smoking, prolonged continual exposure is not necessary. Those exposed to asbestos who smoke are much more likely to develop cancer than those exposed to asbestos who do not smoke.

The problem of exposure in certain jobs is underlined when it is realized that 6 per cent of asbestos workers are known to die of mesothelioma—this is an extremely rare tumour in the normal population. Because of continued industrial exposure over the past 40 years the number of cases is bound to rise further in future years.

Treatment of other lung tumours

DIAGNOSING MESOTHELIOMA

The onset of the tumour is insidious and the most common symptom is a persistent localized chest pain. This is often followed by shortness of breath, tiredness, and discomfort. Fluid usually develops and fills the pleural space (a pleural effusion; see p. 85), although the tumour itself may gradually fill the space between the lung and chest wall. Cough and fever are seen less commonly.

X-rays of the chest may show a plaque of tumour as well as fluid in the pleural space and speckled deposits of calcium (which look like bone) in the pleura.

The diagnosis must be made by obtaining a small piece of tumour for microscopic examination. This may be done using a needle (see p. 35), via a telescope passed into the pleural space (pleuroscopy) or may require a small operation to open up the chest through a space between two ribs.

TREATMENT OF PLEURAL MESOTHELIOMA

Because of the relative rarity of these tumours their treatment has not been studied in large scale trials.

Surgery

Attempts to cure the tumour by extensive operations to remove all the tumour have, unfortunately, met with little success and the operation carries quite a large risk. Despite removal of the pleura and the lung most tumours recur. However, operations designed to reduce symptoms may sometimes be considered.

Radiotherapy

Use of radiotherapy is controversial, with some trials reporting good results and others no benefit at all. Occasional 'cures' have been reported and some patients have had good control of pain but no controlled trials have been done to ascertain just how useful radiotherapy is.

Chemotherapy

Although a small proportion of patients (about one in five) will have a shrinkage of their tumour when treated with anti-cancer drugs, there is

76 Lung cancer: the facts

little evidence of overall benefit because responses are short-lived and there are unpleasant side-effects. Drug treatment should preferably only be used in a trial testing whether new treatments are helpful.

OUTLOOK FOR MESOTHELIOMA

As is the case with most lung tumours, we know the cause of meso-thelioma and the greatest hope for the future lies in recommended tightening of the rules governing the use of asbestos. Implementation of such regulations is all the more important because it is an unfortunate fact that very few patients benefit from current surgery, radiotherapy, or chemotherapy.

RARE TUMOURS OF THE LUNG

As well as the common types of lung cancer there are several rare tumours that may develop in the lungs. Little detailed information is available about most of these, because they are so very rare, and there are often no real guidelines to say what treatment is best.

CARCINOID

This is a special and uncommon type of tumour that generally follows a rather benign course. It develops from cells that usually secrete chemicals (hormones) and some may cause symptoms because of the substances they produce. The small bowel is the most common site for these tumours but occasionally they are found in the lung. Spread to local lymph nodes is found in about 10–20 per cent of patients, and to distant parts of the body in only 5–15 per cent of patients.

The tumour is most common in 50- to 60-year-olds and is rather more frequent in men. Treatment is surgical removal of the tumour whenever possible. If it is too extensive to be removed by an operation, then most will continue to grow slowly and do not spread. Many patients have survived for 10 or more years even though they have not been free of the tumour. Carcinoid tumours that arise in the bowel have a similar, slowly progressive course. Those that begin in the lungs cause fewer symptoms than those of the bowel. These symptoms (flushing, diarrhoea, weakness, facial bloating, etc.) are caused by the release of abnormal amounts of hormones from the tumour.

Treatment of other lung tumours

TRACHEAL CANCER

The trachea is the main airway leading down into the lungs (see Fig. 8, p. 31) and it is surprising that cancer of the trachea is so rare because its structure is similar to the main airways in the lungs. Treatment is usually by radiotherapy, as surgery is not possible. The chances of cure are unfortunately poor because of the central location of the tumour in the chest.

SARCOMAS

These are tumours of the supportive structures in the lungs. Their behaviour is very variable but some are slower growing and have less of a tendency to spread than the common lung cancers. Treatment is by surgery whenever possible, or by radiotherapy.

TUMOURS OF BRONCHIAL GLANDS

Cylindroma is the name given to the most common tumour of the bronchial glands, although it is very rare. Most patients are in their 40s and 50s. The tumour may be slow-growing and both surgery and radiotherapy can be curative.

MIXED TUMOURS OR CARCINOSARCOMAS

These tumours contain a mixture of different tissues. They occur rather earlier (30–40 years of age) than the common lung cancers and spread is seen in about half the patients. They may also be called pulmonary blastomas. Treatment is by surgery or radiotherapy and may be curative.

OTHER TUMOURS

Cancer that spreads from another part of the body to the lungs is very common but should *not* be regarded as a lung cancer or a new tumour. It is a secondary tumour (metastasis) and treatment depends on where the cancer originally developed.

Tumours of the lymph glands (lymphomas, including Hodgkin's disease) may involve or even start in the lungs, but should not be regarded as primary lung cancers. They often respond very well to radiotherapy and chemotherapy (see reading list for further details; p. 118).

10

Other methods of treatment

LASER THERAPY

PHOTORADIATION

In the past few years there has been interest in the use of lasers to treat cancer, and a recent discovery has led to attempts to diagnose lung cancer and subsequently to treat it using a technique known as photoradiation.

A few years ago scientists found that naturally occurring chemicals (called haematoporphyrins) seemed to be absorbed and bound by cancer cells for longer than by normal cells. The chemical itself does not seem to harm the cells but when it is exposed to red light a chemical reaction occurs and the resulting products kill the cell.

Doctors have been using flexible bronchoscopes (see p. 35) to look into the air passages in the lung and it is also possible to use these to transmit a laser beam. Lasers are a powerful source of light and can produce light of particular colours, including the red needed to activate haematoporphyrin. Violet lasers can be used to show up the position of the haematoporphyrin because it causes the chemical to fluoresce, but does not activate it.

Unfortunately, recent data has not confirmed that cancer cells hold on to the haematoporphyrins for longer than normal cells, so this treatment has not proved to be as specific as was hoped.

Detection of cancer using photoradiation

An injection of haematoporphyrin is given and is followed by bronchoscopy when the cancer cells have had time to absorb the chemical. A laser producing a violet light is used to show the cells containing haematoporphyrin.

As haematoporphyrin fluoresces under the violet light the cancer cells show up as a bright fluorescent green area. Theoretically, this technique would be useful for picking up cancers at an early stage, although it does

Other methods of treatment 79

not kill the cancer cells. Because many smokers have precancerous changes in their lungs (see p. 4), it may be possible to detect and treat cancers before they turn malignant. This possibility remains to be tested. The finding of a precancerous change may, however, be enough to persuade a smoker to stop, as there is good evidence that these precancerous changes will regress when the patient stops smoking (see p. 4).

Photoradiation as treatment

Studies of the use of lasers and haematoporphyrin to treat lung cancer have been started recently. After the chemical has been injected and bound by the cancer cells a bronchoscopy is performed using a laser that produces red light. This is shone at the tumour and activates the production of chemicals that cause death of the cancer cell. Once again this technique is in its infancy and, although it sounds very attractive, it is not without its drawbacks.

Complications of photoradiation

Most patients are more sensitive to sunlight for a prolonged period after an injection of haematoporphyrin and sunburn is a common, although generally not a serious, side-effect.

More serious are the local effects of killing the tumour itself. This may lead to quite serious bleeding if the cancer is invading a blood vessel and can result in holes developing in the wall of a major airway if the cancer has invaded through the wall itself.

Because of this, photoradiation should only be used by those experienced in the technique and preferably in trials testing whether it has a useful role in the care of lung cancer. If it is used it must be remembered that other treatments often fail because tumour spread has already occurred; photoradiation will not overcome these problems because it is a purely local treatment.

LASER SURGERY

A simpler use of lasers is to use them to cut through tumour that is blocking a major airway. This can be useful in selected patients, for example to open up a blocked lung. It is more likely that laser therapy will find a role when used this way, rather than in photoradiation.

80 Lung cancer: the facts

INTERNAL IRRADIATION

Radioactive sources can be implanted inside the body so that they are in contact with a tumour, thus delivering a high dose of irradiation. Although this technique has been routinely used for some years against tumours such as occur in cervical cancer, it is only recently that this technique has been used in lung cancer.

A thin tube is passed into the airway using a flexible bronchoscope (p. 35) and using a device called a microselectron a radioactive source is briefly introduced into the lung to treat the tumour. This technique is an alternative to laser therapy and can unblock an airway full of tumour.

HEAT AS A TREATMENT FOR LUNG CANCER (HYPERTHERMIA)

Scientists have known for many years that cancer cells seem to be more sensitive to heat than normal ones; indeed during the last century cancer was sometimes treated by inoculating patients with toxins that caused a high fever.

If a tumour is heated up to 41–43 °C (normal body temperature is 37 °C) then cancer cells are frequently killed or seriously damaged, whilst normal cells are unaffected. The situation is, in fact, rather more complicated than this as it is only the poorly nourished cancer cells in the centre of the tumour that are affected (Fig. 15). Nearly all cancers seem to outgrow their blood supply and there are areas that are acidic and have too little oxygen; it seems that these cells are the ones most sensitive to heat. This is very convenient, as these are the cells that are most insensitive to radiation because of low oxygen concentrations (oxygen is needed for radiation to work) and to drugs because of poor spread of anti-cancer drugs into the cancer.

However, hyperthermia is only now being studied scientifically and it is too early to say whether it will be useful in lung cancer. There are two main approaches; it may be possible to heat the tumour itself, or to heat the whole patient. Clearly it is easier to heat part of body, especially if there is, say, tumour in a limb, than to heat the whole patient to a high temperature for some hours.

Early results suggest that some tumours may shrink if treated locally and a variety of machines are available to do this. It also seems that such

Other methods of treatment

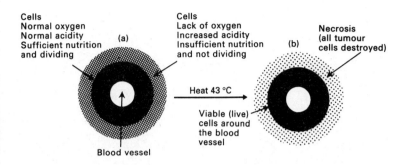

Fig. 15 Hyperthermia. (a) Cells nearest to the blood vessel are healthy; those furthest away are not. (b) The unhealthy cells furthest from the blood vessel are destroyed when the tumour is heated.

treatment is more effective if given together with radiation or chemotherapy, as the various treatments kill different cells in the tumour.

Heating the whole body must be done in a very carefully controlled way as it puts a strain on the heart, lungs, and blood vessels. If hyperthermia is to prove useful in lung cancer, some form of whole-body heating is likely to be needed because of the inaccessibility of the tumour and the high likelihood of tumour spread. Until trials show whether it is effective, hyperthermia should only be used in closely monitored trials.

11

Treatment of the symptoms and complications of lung cancer

Many patients will have symptoms from their lung cancer when they first see their doctor, or may develop symptoms later if the tumour is not controlled. This section outlines some of the problems that can arise and discusses how they are treated, although it is important to remember that many patients will develop only a few of these symptoms. Of course, the best treatment for any symptom is to get rid of the underlying cause —the cancer. However, even if this is not possible for some patients, there are many ways in which symptoms can be reduced to improve a patient's life.

LUNG COLLAPSE

Lung cancers, because they grow in the main airways, may obstruct the air passages supplying part or all of a lung (Fig. 16). The severity of symptoms produced will depend on the amount of lung that is affected. Early symptoms include cough, haemoptysis (coughing up blood), shortness of breath on exertion, and wheezing. If the obstruction becomes complete a persistent cough, with or without blood in the sputum, may develop and chest discomfort, shortness of breath and wheeze may become more severe. Infection often develops in the collapsed part of the lung and this will cause fevers and chills, loss of appetite and weight, and general malaise. This should be treated with antibiotics regardless of other therapies.

Ideally, treatment is given to shrink the tumour so that the blockage is removed. Radiotherapy (see p. 58) can be very effective, although it should be remembered that it is usually not possible to use radiotherapy more than once, as it will cause unacceptable damage to normal tissues. Chemotherapy (see p. 67) can be helpful in some tumours although the side-effects of treatment must be weighed carefully against the benefits in non-small-cell lung cancer. Lasers (see p. 78), with or without haemato-

Treatment of the symptoms and complications

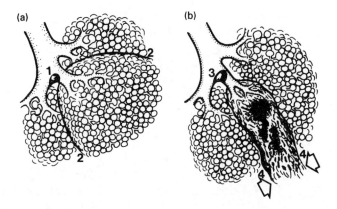

Fig. 16 Collapse of a segment of the lung. (a) A tumour (1) starts to grow in the airway supplying a segment of lung that is bordered by fibrous bands (2). (b) The tumour (3) grows and nearly completely blocks the airway to the segment. This results in collapse (see arrows) of the fibrous borders (4) of the segment and infection.

porphyrins, and internal radiotherapy (see p. 80) have been used in some patients to reduce blockage of an airway, but these techniques are only available in some hospitals.

If it is not possible to give treatment to remove the blockage, then treatment should be directed at removing troublesome symptoms such as cough (p. 92), infection, and pain (p. 93).

VENOUS OBSTRUCTION

A large tumour growing in the centre of the chest may press on the major veins as they are about to enter the heart (Fig. 17). This large vein (the superior vena cava) drains blood from the head, neck, arms, and upper chest. Any significant pressure on the vein will slow down the blood drainage and all the veins in the area that should be drained will become overfull and distended. This results in swelling of the face, neck, and upper chest and arms. Veins in these area frequently become more visible than normal.

Ideally, treatment is given to shrink the tumour and relieve the pressure. Radiotherapy is usually the most effective treatment, although

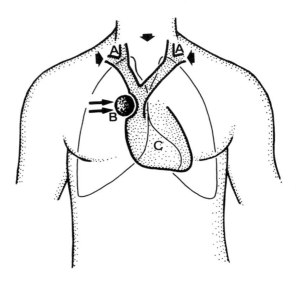

Fig. 17 Superior vena caval obstruction. The blood from the neck and arms drains into the main veins in the chest (short arrows and A). A tumour (B) pressing on the main vein (the superior vena cava) before it enters the heart (C) will block the blood vessel causing back pressure and swelling of the neck, arms, and face.

in the case of small-cell lung cancer, chemotherapy may be used first. Steroids may also be used to try to reduce the amount of oedema and swelling. If radiotherapy has been used and cannot be repeated, chemotherapy and/or steroids may help reduce the pressure on the superior vena cava.

PLEURAL EFFUSION

A pleural effusion is a collection of fluid between the chest wall and the lung. Because it compresses the lung it will cause shortness of breath as it gets larger (Fig. 18).

It is a relatively simple procedure to remove the fluid from a pleural effusion that has become large enough to cause troublesome breathlessness. For patients who have not had problems from the effusion before, it may be enough to push a thin needle through the chest wall into the fluid

Treatment of the symptoms and complications

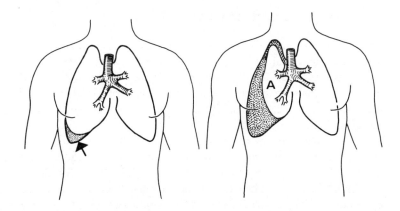

Fig. 18 Pleural effusion. This starts as a small collection of fluid (arrow) between the lung and chest wall. If it increases it may gradually fill the pleural space on the side of the chest, compressing the lung (A).

and then suck it off. This is done under a local anaesthetic and is quite quick. As the fluid is being removed, the changing position of the lung may cause some discomfort and coughing. If the procedure becomes uncomfortable, tell the doctor as this is often an indication to stop because nearly all the fluid has been removed. A chest X-ray will be taken after the procedure (called a pleurocentesis) to check that the fluid has gone and that no air has been allowed to leak into the pleural space (a pneumothorax).

If the fluid keeps coming back despite pleurocentesis, a minor operation may be done (under local anaesthetic) to pass a thin tube into the pleural fluid. This is left in place and is connected to a sealed water bottle (see p. 54). If necessary this may be connected to a pump that sucks out as much fluid as possible. When the pleural space is as 'dry' as possible a drug may be injected through the tube to produce inflammation of the surfaces of the pleura in an attempt to produce scar tissue that will seal off the pleural space. If this succeeds it will prevent the formation of a new effusion. Although the chest tube and drug both cause discomfort and require the patient to come into hospital for a day or two, the chances of success are about 50:50 so it is well worth trying if a pleural effusion keeps coming back. The type of drug injected through the tube varies, and some may cause a temporary burning discomfort or a fever, which can be helped by anti-inflammatory pain killers such as aspirin.

PERICARDIAL EFFUSION

The heart is surrounded by a sac—the pericardium—which may fill with fluid, much as pleural fluid can fill the space between the chest wall and lungs (see p. 84). Because this sac is not very flexible, the fluid quickly fills it and starts to exert pressure on the beating heart. If the amount of fluid continues to increase it eventually affects the heart's pumping action, so that it starts to fail.

Because of the pressure the heart is not able to fill with blood properly and the back pressure causes fluid to build up in the lungs, and eventually in the body tissues. This results in increasing shortness of breath and swelling of the ankles. The blood pressure often falls and this causes the patient to feel dizzy, especially on suddenly standing up. These symptoms can be caused by many other things, changes in heart rhythm for instance, but if fluid is shown to be building up around the heart it often needs to be removed. The diagnosis of a pericardial effusion is made on clinical examination by a doctor and is confirmed by ultrasound examination of the heart. The usual cause of pericardial effusion in lung cancer is direct invasion of the cancer into the pericardium around the heart.

If a significant amount of fluid is found to be affecting the heart's action, the effusion must be drained. After an injection of local anaesthetic, a thin needle is passed between the ribs and carefully pushed forwards until it is in the fluid around the heart, which is then sucked out. Although this sounds a very difficult and hazardous procedure, it is in fact relatively easy to do. To reduce any risks the needle is connected to an electrocardiogram (ECG) machine and this shows, on a television screen, if the tip of the needle touches the heart itself. Provided that treatment can be given to control the tumour that is causing the build-up of fluid, this may be all that is necessary.

However, if fluid keeps building up it may become necessary to do a small operation to remove a portion (called a window) of the front of the pericardial sac. This allows the fluid to drain into the chest, where it is less of a problem. It is also possible to inject a drug into the pericardial sac in an attempt to try to stop the fluid coming back.

HORMONE PRODUCTION BY LUNG CANCERS

Any malignant tumour can produce hormones (chemical messengers that control the body's glands and some of its functions) but lung

Treatment of the symptoms and complications   87

tumours do so more often than any other type of cancer. Normally the amounts of various hormones in the body are very carefully regulated by a variety of delicate checks and balances. However, when a tumour produces a hormone it ignores these checks and balances and excessive amounts of the hormone are secreted into the bloodstream. The vast excess of the hormone causes abnormal changes in the body, the nature of which depend on the type of hormone being produced. Some of the more common problems are outlined below.

CORTICOSTEROID (CORTISOL) EXCESS

Some lung tumours may secrete a hormone called ACTH, whose normal job is to stimulate the adrenal glands to produce steroid hormones. These will have a number of effects, which include:

- increased weight;
- deposition of fat over the face and trunk but not the limbs; this produces a round face (sometimes called a moonface) and a fat pad over the shoulders;
- muscle weakness, which may become severe;
- changes in the balance of salts (especially potassium in the blood) and a raised blood pressure.

The best way to treat this condition is to deal with the underlying cause—the tumour. If surgery, radiotherapy, or chemotherapy can shrink or get rid of the cancer, this relieves the symptoms. Drugs that block the production of the steroid hormones in the adrenal gland can be tried but control of the cancer is the only sure way to prevent the symptoms.

EXCESS ANTIDIURETIC HORMONE (ADH)

This hormone is normally concerned in controlling how much water the kidneys retain in the body; it is frequently produced in small-cell lung cancer (see p. 8). Symptoms of excess production (known as the syndrome of inappropriate anti-diuretic hormone or SIADH) include:

- loss of appetite;
- nausea and vomiting;
- lethargy;
- abnormal levels of salts in the blood (low sodium).

88 Lung cancer: the facts

Treatment is preferably that of the underlying tumour that is over-producing the hormone (ADH). Because it is most commonly associated with small-cell cancers this may be possible with chemotherapy, even when the tumour is widespread. Whilst treatment is being started, simple restriction of fluid intake, below 1 litre a day, or the use of an antibiotic that interferes with the salt/water balance (demeclocycline) can improve the symptoms. It is very important to maintain the strict fluid intake because excess fluids can make the patient very unwell and can even lead to fits caused by the brain becoming waterlogged.

EXCESS CALCIUM IN BLOOD (HYPERCALCAEMIA)

This is particularly common in squamous lung cancer (see p. 7) and may be due to the overproduction of a hormone similar to parathyroid hormone by the tumour—this hormone controls the balance of calcium in the blood and the bones. Less commonly it may arise because there is extensive tumour in bones that releases calcium. The symptoms are:

- loss of appetite;
- nausea;
- excessive thirst and excessive urine production;
- constipation;
- drowsiness that can lead to near-coma.

Treatment is, as in similar situations, that of the underlying tumour. Whilst treatment is being started the symptoms may be helped by a high fluid intake (by an infusion into a vein if necessary) and use of some new drugs that control calcium—pamidronate or etidronate. Judicious use of the measures should control the symptoms in nearly all patients.

OTHER HORMONE SYNDROMES

Many other different types of hormones may be produced by lung cancers but this is relatively uncommon.

SPREAD OF LUNG CANCER TO THE BONES

Spread of lung cancer to the bones is unfortunately fairly common late in the course of the disease. Pain is the most frequent symptom. Because

Treatment of the symptoms and complications   89

the bones are weakened by the tumour, breaks or fractures can occur after even minor injury.

Treatment is primarily radiotherapy to the painful bone or fracture, although some fractures in bones in the arms or legs will need special support. This usually means a small operation to put a steel pin down the centre of the bone to give it stability. Radiotherapy is usually very good at relieving bone pain but pain-killing medicines may sometimes be necessary. Anti-inflammatory drugs like aspirin seem to be particularly good at reducing bone pain and can be added to other pain-killing drugs.

Swelling of the bones at the fingertips together with curvature of the nails (clubbing) is quite common in lung cancer. In some patients this may progress to painful swellings at various joints, called hypertrophic pulmonary osteoarthropathy. The only way of improving these is successful treatment of the cancer itself, which suggests that it is caused by something produced by the cancer. If it is not possible to shrink the cancer, anti-inflammatory pain killers and sometimes steroids can be used to reduce the discomfort.

SPREAD OF LUNG CANCER TO THE BRAIN OR NERVES

BRAIN

The idea of a tumour affecting the brain is terrifying because it seems to attack the centre of our very being. Unfortunately, lung cancers can spread to the brain and cause all sorts of different symptoms. Fortunately, these can often be controlled and only occur in a minority of patients. Spread to the brain is most often seen in small-cell lung cancer and is more common when patients have responded well to their treatment and have lived for longer periods. This allows the tumour the chance to grow in the brain, the one place where the drugs may not have reached (see p. 71). For this reason, some patients with small-cell lung cancer receive brain radiotherapy after initial chemotherapy in an attempt to prevent the tumour growing (prophylactic cranial irradiation).

If a tumour does affect the brain, it can produce many different symptoms according to which part of the brain is affected. The common symptoms are:

- severe headache—usually worse on waking and made worse by straining or coughing;

90 Lung cancer: the facts

- nausea and vomiting;
- weakness of part of the body;
- change of feeling in part of the body;
- disturbance in balance;
- disturbance of vision;
- change in mood;
- fits, as in epilepsy.

If spread of lung cancer to the brain is found, usually by a CT scan (see p. 44), radiotherapy is generally given; surgery is very rarely, if ever, indicated. Steroid treatment with the drug dexamethasone is often used first, to reduce any inflammation and swelling (oedema) around the tumour. Because the brain is enclosed in the bony skull, any swelling rapidly causes pressure on the brain, which causes headache and other symptoms. Dexamethasone usually relieves this promptly and reduces the symptoms. If a fit has occurred, anti-epileptic drugs—generally phenobarbitone and phenytoin—will be given to prevent any more.

Radiotherapy shrinks the tumour and anti-cancer drug therapy is rarely required. Although the response is often dramatic, it is unfortunately often temporary, although it is very useful in reducing symptoms.

SPINAL CORD

Occasionally a lung tumour may spread to affect the spinal cord rather than the brain. This will cause:

- weakness, usually in both legs;
- loss or change in sensation in the lower part of the body—the upper level of this loss of feeling depending on the site of the tumour;
- disturbed bowel and bladder function so that normal control is lost.

Anyone with these symptoms should see a doctor *immediately*, as it is of the utmost urgency that treatment is started early. Symptoms which are allowed to progress may become permanent. If an early operation (to relieve the pressure on the spine) or radiotherapy is given then there is a chance of full recovery. Dexamethasone should be started as soon as the diagnosis is suspected to reduce any swelling and oedema. Patients with the symptoms or signs of pressure on the spinal cord should be referred to a neurosurgeon or radiotherapist immediately; undue delay risks permanent loss of power in the legs with loss of bowel and bladder function (paraplegia).

Treatment of the symptoms and complications 91

NERVES

Pressure from the tumour on a nerve will damage it and often stop it working normally. The most common places for this to happen in patients with lung cancer are in the centre of the chest and in the neck. The nerve to the left side of the larynx loops down into the chest near the heart and a tumour involving lymph glands in the left side of the chest may press on it, causing marked hoarseness. This is because the left-hand vocal cord no longer receives messages from the brain and cannot move. An injection of Teflon directly into the vocal cord can be used to try to improve the hoarseness but there is rarely any treatment that will cause the nerve to start working normally after it has been damaged.

Similarly, when tumours develop in the top part of the lung (superior sulcus tumours; see p. 64), they may affect a special nerve that supplies the eye. This will cause drooping of the eyelid on that side, a contracted pupil, and a slightly depressed eyeball—a condition known as Horner's syndrome. Although it is not dangerous in itself it is troublesome, as it responds poorly to treatment even if the tumour shrinks. Tumours in this area can also involve the complex sheath of nerves supplying the arm (the brachial plexus) and pressure can lead to pain, weakness, and altered sensation.

GENERALIZED EFFECTS ON THE NERVES AND BRAIN

A few patients develop symptoms, often before there is any sign of lung cancer, that cannot be explained by the presence of cancer pressing on, or directly infiltrating, the nervous system. These symptoms may improve when the cancer is treated and it is believed that such symptoms are caused by chemicals that damage the nervous system—the chemicals being produced by the tumour itself.

The common symptoms are:

- weakness of muscles;
- loss of balance;
- change in sensation or feeling;
- muscle weakness and pain with wasting of the muscles.

These sorts of symptoms are very general in their nature and are very common, so that it is important to remember that only very rarely are they due to a developing lung cancer.

92   Lung cancer: the facts

SKIN RASHES

Occasionally a cancer that starts in the lung may grow through the chest wall and appear as a nodular area in the skin. This raised area is often purplish, can form an ulcer and bleed, and may be uncomfortable. Radiotherapy or chemotherapy may be able to shrink it down and pain-killers may be needed. There is no danger of severe bleeding.

Some patients with cancer may develop skin changes that are not directly caused by invasion of the skin by the tumour. It seems likely that they are caused by chemicals produced by the tumour itself, as they tend to improve when the cancer is removed. There are a wide variety of these skin rashes, although they are all rather uncommon. Some patients develop extensive dark pigmented areas, especially under the arms, whilst others have scaly or blistered areas. Occasionally these rashes may be associated with muscle pain and weakness (a condition called dermatomyositis). Most patients with lung cancer do not have one of these syndromes, and certainly anyone with a rash is very unlikely to turn out to have cancer.

Treatment of the underlying cancer is the surest way to improve the rash, although steroids can be helpful, particularly if muscle pains and weakness are present.

COUGH

A cough is the most common symptom caused by lung cancer and can be continuous and very trying. Any treatment that can get rid of the cancer itself is the best way of dealing with it. However, if this is not possible it can usually be helped with various cough suppressants. These, in increasing strength, include:

- codeine linctus;
- pholcodine linctus;
- methadone linctus;
- diamorphine linctus.

Other types of cough medicine may be used:

- expectorants that stimulate the cough to try to help clear the lung secretion;

Treatment of the symptoms and complications 93

- mucolytics, designed to reduce the thickness of any phlegm so that it is brought up more easily.

For most patients a cough suppressant is all that is required, although a mucolytic may be helpful in some patients.

PAIN

Many people think of cancer as a fatal disease in which pain is always a problem. In fact, about a half of patients with advancing cancer do not have significant pain but, for those who do, expert care can ensure that it is kept under control. It is also worth remembering that patients with cancer can be cured, and that this applies even to lung cancer, although it is often a difficult tumour to treat.

Pain in lung cancer is most commonly due to invasion into the chest wall or sensitive structures in the chest or spread of tumour into the bones. If radiotherapy or chemotherapy can be used to shrink the tumour, this is obviously the best way of dealing with the problem. If this is not possible, appropriate use of pain killers and other drugs can control most of the pain and discomfort.

Pain often varies in severity during the day and is usually worse at night. This may be partly due to the use of drugs that ease pain for a while and then allow it to return, although it is also largely related to mood. Pain is not just a simple physical sensation, it is very greatly influenced and made worse by depression, anxiety, and all sorts of stress. Chronic pain can take over one's life, if it:

- seems to be without a foreseeable end;
- tends to get worse rather than better;
- serves no purpose;
- takes up all your attention and can make life not seem worth living.

This type of pain needs expert treatment and in most cases can be controlled, making life worthwhile again.

USING PAIN-KILLERS

The essence of controlling pain is to give an effective dose of a pain-killer often enough to keep the pain at bay at all times. This sounds obvious, but all too often patients, doctors, and nurses are reluctant to use

94   Lung cancer: the facts

frequent doses of strong pain-killers. It is never helpful to use pain-killers only when the pain is bad; this tends to lead to gradually increasing doses to control the worsening pain.

For instance, if after taking a pain-killer a patient is pain-free for 4½–5 hours they will need to take the next dose after 4 hours, so that the drug has been fully absorbed before the pain returns. It is best to give pain-killers by mouth and injections can be avoided in nearly all patients. It is important to remember that, when powerful pain-killers are being used to control pain addiction is not a real problem. Regular doses of drugs like morphine and heroin (known as diamorphine) may be taken safely.

Unless pain is very severe it is best to start with simple pain-killers and to increase the strength gradually until the pain is controlled. Some of the drugs used are shown below but many others are also available.

Mild pain

This is usually well treated by aspirin or paracetamol (Panadol). One or two tablets should be taken every 4 hours.

Moderate pain

If aspirin or paracetamol are insufficient, weak narcotic drugs can be used. These often contain a combination of drugs, usually including codeine. The commonly prescribed drugs are:

- Co-proxamol (paracetamol and dextropropoxyphene);
- Codis (aspirin and codeine);
- Paracodol (paracetamol and codeine);
- DF118 (dihydrocodeine);
- Paramol 118 (paracetamol and dihydrocodeine).

The usual dose is one or two tablets every four hours. There are many other similar drugs; all require a doctor's prescription.

Severe pain

Stronger narcotic drugs are usually needed and can be given safely and regularly and are always worth trying. The dose can often be reduced once the pain is under control. Some may cause sleepiness and loss of concentration is common at first, although this gradually improves as the body gets used to the pain-killer. Fortunately, the pain continues to

Treatment of the symptoms and complications   95

be controlled by the same dose and increasing doses are not normally needed once the right dose has been found. Available drugs include:

- Nepenthe (with or without aspirin), a mixture of opium alkaloids with morphine;
- MST Continus: a slow-release morphine with the advantage that it only need be taken twice a day;
- morphine syrup;
- diamorphine;
- phenazocine (Narphen): an alternative to diamorphine that causes less nausea, but that is not available in liquid form;
- buprenorphine (Temgesic): a moderately strong narcotic that can be sucked under the tongue.

These drugs are best given by mouth on a regular basis. If a patient wakes with pain at night it is sometimes worth setting an alarm clock to wake before the pain returns, as it is easier to go back to sleep whilst still relatively pain-free than it is when the pain has returned.

In the past, narcotic drugs were often mixed together with other drugs and alcohol to form a cocktail, drugs such as anti-depressants or anti-anxiety drugs can be used separately with pain-killers when they are needed. If they are used separately then the doses of each can be more carefully controlled.

Pain is much worse if depression or stress is a problem and the use of appropriate drugs to deal with depression and anxiety are very helpful in getting pain under control. When bone or nerve pain is a problem anti-inflammatory drugs can be very helpful in addition to the ordinary pain-killers.

Perhaps one of the most important ways doctors, nurses, and families can help the patient with pain is to take the time to listen to them. Isolation and depression make it much more difficult to control the pain and half an hour spent listening to and talking with a patient may mean that the efficacy of a drug is greatly increased.

OTHER WAYS OF STOPPING PAIN

If drugs are ineffective, other methods can be tried.

Nerve blocks

Because pain sensations are carried by nerves, anything that damages nerves and blocks their ability to carry messages can reduce the feeling of

96   Lung cancer: the facts

pain. Injections of local anaesthetic or substances designed to damage nerves can be given. They can be helpful in particular cases, although in some instances there is a risk that they may damage the function of the part of the body supplied by the nerve that has been injected. Because of this it is important to discuss with the doctor the advantages and disadvantages of such treatment. Nerve blocks are usually only available in special pain clinics.

Transcutaneous nerve stimulation (TNS)

Electrical stimulation of skin near a painful area may reduce the pain itself. Unfortunately the effect is usually quite temporary.

Hypnosis

This can be used together with other methods of pain control but is usually only of temporary benefit. Its main value may be that the doctor spends half an hour with the patient.

Acupuncture

This seems to give temporary relief of pain to some patients, but has so far been little used in cancer patients.

The important features of pain control are:

- Pain is not only physical; treatment of depression and anxiety or even just the opportunity to discuss their illness and feelings is a great help to most patients.
- Severe pain can nearly always be, at least partially, controlled.
- A strong-enough drug must be used regularly so that unacceptable pain does not return between doses.
- Narcotic drugs do not cause addiction if used to control pain.
- Other methods are available if drugs do not work.

LOSS OF APPETITE AND WEIGHT

This is very common when a patient has a growing tumour and may be due to several factors:

Treatment of the symptoms and complications   97

- The tumour may be altering the body's metabolism and burning up excessive amounts of energy.
- The tumour and its treatment may be causing nausea and vomiting, diarrhoea or failure to absorb food that is eaten.
- Tumours sometimes cause patients to feel revolted by the sight or smell of food—they just do not feel like eating.
- Anxiety.

Prolonged loss of appetite, called anorexia, leads to wasting, which is known as cachexia. This is difficult to treat as the more weight a patient loses, the less they feel like eating. Family and friends are concerned and often press the patient to eat, which usually only makes things worse.

It is best for a patient to try to eat small regular meals of anything that they fancy. Foods with a strong smell should be avoided and things that look attractive should be chosen. A drink of alcohol or a tonic before eating may help but the use of steroids (prednisone or dexamethasone) is usually the surest way of improving appetite. Prednisone, in addition to improving appetite, usually gives a general feeling of well-being. Alternatively, megestrol acetate (a hormone used to treat breast cancer) may be used to stimulate appetite—it has the advantage of not causing the side-effects of steroids.

Food supplements can be helpful and supply calories and protein. The main problem is that it is often difficult to find a flavour that is palatable. It is often worth trying a sample of different flavours of various food supplements to see if there is one that is more palatable than the others.

12
Talking about lung cancer

For most people cancer is a dreaded disease and cancer of the lung is particularly feared. Because of this, it has become a subject shrouded in secrecy and mystery. Doctors often feel unable to talk to patients about their illness and treatment, and those who were cured have failed to tell others, which has perpetuated the myth that everyone dies. If you have read the rest of this book you will have found that, unfortunately, very many patients with lung cancer *do* die of their tumour, but there are some who are cured and many others who benefit from treatment. Although doctors have traditionally been slow to acknowledge that many patients want to know what is happening to them, they are coming to realize that most patients want to know about their illness and treatment—even if the news is not good.

For the majority it is a great help to know what they are facing; for about three-quarters it is only confirmation of what they already feared, and an imagined situation is often more frightening than the truth. When a patient has not been told, but their close family has, a very destructive situation can arise where no-one can discuss what is happening for fear of causing distress, although everyone, including the patient, knows what is happening. This situation causes unimaginable tension and often results from a request from the patient or family not to discuss the diagnosis openly, or even because the doctor feels that the patient should not know—although the family is told. So, although everyone is trying to be kind, these good intentions usually cause more pain than the simple truth.

In most situations a straightforward explanation of the disease and its treatment, preferably given to both the patient and their family at the same time, is helpful. Any questions should be answered with honesty, tempered with sensitivity. If there is good information as well as bad, this should be given as soon as possible in a realistic manner.

It is very important for patients to develop a good relationship with doctors and nurses and, as mentioned before, this book is intended only to be a back-up to this. I hope that it will help to develop open discussion

Talking about lung cancer

by prompting questions as well as providing practical information and sources of help.

Once the diagnosis of lung cancer is out in the open it is then possible to discuss how it is going to be handled. Discussions about tests, treatment, and the outlook will hopefully proceed at a pace that the patient can handle comfortably: if patients are allowed to lead the discussion this is ensured. Family, doctors, and nurses need to learn to *listen* to patients, their frustrations, worries, and questions. Anyone with cancer is under severe stress from the first time they realize what the trouble may be, and they will continue to have emotional ups and downs during the course of the disease.

FINDING OUT WHAT IS WRONG

Very often, discovering a symptom (such as coughing up blood) that suggests cancer to the individual can be even more shocking than actually finding out that it *is* cancer. The seriousness of the potential situation is often not helped by the doctor's uncomfortable silence and everyone's reluctance to discuss what it might be. Patients not infrequently say that this was their lowest period—when they felt most alone, and even if they confide their fears everyone understandably tries to give false reassurance. Often it may be several weeks before the diagnosis is known and by then patients are often so worried that they feel unable to ask what it is, unless their doctor 'gives them permission', and a conspiracy of silence develops.

Once the diagnosis is confirmed a series of staging tests (see p. 38) is done and all too often no explanation is given and patients feel pushed from pillar to post. A simple explanation of what tests will be done, how they are to be done, and why they are necessary makes life so much easier. Even when an explanation is given, many patients are so shocked and upset that they are able to take very little in and a simple fact-sheet explaining the tests may be helpful.

Patients who want to know should ask about the tests and, if they want to know the results, they have every right to request these. One of the biggest crises for patients with cancer is loss of control of their own life. Suddenly struck with cancer, they are taken over by the hospital and seemingly have no power over their destiny. Inclusion of those patients who wish it into the whole process of diagnosis and treatment goes a

100　　　　　　Lung cancer: the facts

good way to reducing their feeling of helplessness. Patients who want to ask questions may find it helpful to write them down; it is only too easy to forget what they were during the stress of seeing the doctor.

Support organizations, such as Cancer Link and BACUP, can answer many questions for patients and their families. They can also supply much relevant information, including details on support groups, etc. These and other organizations (see Appendix) are listed at the back of the book with appropriate addresses and telephone numbers.

Part 3 The future

13
Clinical trials

Before it can be widely used a new medical or surgical treatment has to be tested to see if it is effective. The only way to do this is to try the treatment out on patients once it has passed extensive safety tests. Although trials of new methods of surgery, radiotherapy, and novel treatments such as hyperthermia (see p. 80) are done, the testing of new drug therapy (chemotherapy) provides the best example of how trials are run.

Many patients, understandably, worry about the possibility of being experimented on, although appreciating that new treatments have to be tested. However, the possibility of inclusion in a proper trial of a new treatment is much better than the alternative of allowing new treatments to be tried without proper organization. In a well-run trial a patient should:

- be told that they are being considered for inclusion in the trial;
- be informed about their illness;
- be given full details about the possible treatments to be used in the trial;
- be told of any other treatments that are available;
- be told of any side-effects they may encounter;
- have the option to agree to be included in the study or elect not to, without any prejudice to further care.

INFORMED CONSENT

Recently the idea that patients should know all about their illness and the trial so that they may make an informed decision about whether they agree to the trial has become accepted. In some countries this means that there is a legal obligation on the part of the doctor to explain the trial and to provide written details (a fact-sheet) prior to asking the patient to give their consent in writing. Although there is no such legal requirement in the United Kingdom there is a movement in this direction. If you think that your treatment could be part of a trial, then you have every right to ask if this is so. If it is, you should ask for full details including:

104 Lung cancer: the facts

- what are the possible benefits?
- what are the risks?
- how is the treatment given?
- what is known about the new treatment?
- will it be compared with another treatment?
- if it is, will I be able to make the choice or will it be by chance?
- will I need to come into hospital for the treatment?
- will I need any other tests that would not normally be done?
- how long will the trial go on for?

If you do take part in a trial you must do so voluntarily, having had all your questions answered to your satisfaction. Do not feel that you need to make a decision the first time you are asked—if you need time to think about it, say so.

Remember that there are many safeguards for patients. Each trial must be approved an an Ethics Committee, composed of doctors, nurses, scientists, and lay people. It is their job to ensure that the trial is scientifically sound, well designed, properly run, and ethical. As well as any benefit from new treatment, you may gain from the extra attention that you will probably receive because of the trial.

Although 'informed consent' sounds like a good idea, it is worth remembering that it takes years to train a doctor, so that very few patients really know 'all about' their illness and its treatment. There must, therefore, always be an element of trust between patient and doctor in a trial.

DIFFERENT TYPES OF TRIAL

Trials are designed to answer different questions, and because of this they are run in various ways. Trials of drug therapy may be of the following kinds:

PHASE I TRIALS

The aim of this type of trial is to see what the side-effects of the new treatment are and what dose is safe. Although extensive laboratory tests will have been done to learn about potential side-effects, this is the first time it will have been used in patients, so there are some risks attached to this type of trial. In addition, no-one knows whether the new treatment will work.

Clinical trials 105

Because of this, phase I trials are only done in patients for whom there is no other known alternative treatment. The chances of benefit for the patients are very small and there will nearly always be some side-effects. Patients should therefore think very carefully before agreeing to these trials; they offer a small hope, but it is more realistic to say they benefit other patients in the future.

PHASE II TRIALS

At this stage doctors know about most of the side-effects, have arrived at a safe dose, and are now trying to determine whether the new treatment has a useful anti-cancer effect. Because its effectiveness is unknown it is only ethical to use the treatment in patients who have no other alternative useful treatment available to them. The chances that the treatment will be very beneficial are not very good, but every so often a very active drug is found in such studies. Most of these trials do not compare treatments and are not randomized (treatment chosen by chance—see below).

PHASE III AND IV TRIALS

When a new treatment has been shown to have a useful anti-cancer effect in phase II trials it will be compared with existing treatments in a phase III and IV trials. In many of these it is necessary to select which treatment is to be given to each patient by chance (randomization) so there is no bias to one type of treatment. Only when a patient has agreed to join in the trial is the treatment selected. Neither the doctor nor patient will know which treatment is going to be picked—so both treatments must be acceptable to the patient.

Because the treatment will have been shown to be active in a phase II study the chances of benefit are much better, although only the trial can decide if the new treatment is a real advance.

At present, very few patients with lung cancer are treated in a trial and more new trials are undoubtedly needed. However, it is essential that patients have confidence in the trial and their doctor. Remember, even if you do start treatment in a trial you may withdraw from it at any time and this will not affect your care at all.

14

Future prospects in lung cancer

PREVENTION

The good news about lung cancer is that we are at last starting to win the battle to prevent future cases. Recently published figures (Office of Population Censuses and Surveys, 1990) show that the number of smokers in the United Kingdom is falling. From 1972 to 1990 the proportion of men smoking fell from 52 per cent to 32 per cent. For women, the fall in the same time period, was from 41 per cent to 28 per cent. As well as more men stopping smoking, those men who continued smoked less; unfortunately there has been little change in the number of cigarettes smoked by those women who have continued.

Happily the number of young men who start smoking is at last falling, although it is worrying that smoking is now as common amongst young women as young men. There is, however, no doubt that the serious consequences of smoking are well known and this has resulted in 1 in 4 smokers giving up in the last 20 years. This may well mean that in 10–20 years time there will be 4000 to 5000 fewer people a year dying from lung cancer.

Whilst low-tar cigarettes and tobacco substitutes may be helpful (see p. 18), the only sure way of combating all of the diseases associated with smoking is to persuade people that smoking is socially and medically undesirable. Although a truism, it is clear that smokers can only stop when the need to stop is stronger than the need to continue. For many long-term smokers this may never happen, but young people are starting to feel that there is not enough to be gained from smoking to make the financial and health costs worth it.

EARLY DIAGNOSIS AND SCREENING

Whilst the early diagnosis of any cancer makes good sense, we do not have sufficiently sensitive tests to diagnose lung cancer before it has

Future prospects in lung cancer 107

spread. Until it has been shown in a trial that the diagnosis can be made early enough to ensure that people are more likely to be cured, there is little point in trying to screen for lung cancer.

TESTS LOOKING FOR SPREAD OF LUNG CANCER (STAGING)

If non-small-cell lung cancer has been diagnosed, then tests are done to see if an operation to remove the tumour will be beneficial (see p. 49). Staging is important, as extensive spread within or outside the chest will mean that an operation will be unhelpful. New tests, such as CT scanning and possibly magnetic resonance image (MRI) scanning, mean that we will be able to localize tumours more efficiently.

Antibodies are proteins produced by the body's immune system as defensive response to infection and the presence of substances not normally found in the body. For instance, antibodies may be produced to attack bacteria that are invading the body. Each antibody is specific for one foreign protein and will only attack that particular protein. Antibodies directed against tumour cells can be made and linked to radioisotopes. This can be used to make images of the tumour with a gamma camera (see p. 41), which produces a picture showing where the antibody–isotope complex sticks to the cancer cells. These techniques may allow better selection of patients for operation. In the case of small-cell lung cancer they will allow more accurate definition of the extent of the tumour and may help to select treatment if radiotherapy or surgery is included.

TREATMENT

SURGERY

It is unlikely that new or better operations will be devised for the treatment of lung cancer; the limiting factor is the early spread of the tumour. Improved selection of patients for operation (see p. 49) will mean that fewer unnecessary operations will be done. For localized non-small-cell lung cancer an operation remains the most effective treatment and continued improvement in post-operative care will reduce the risks from operation. Surgery is less commonly used as the first treatment in small-cell lung cancer and, when it is, it should be combined with chemo-

108 Lung cancer: the facts

therapy. Patients with small-cell cancer, who have responded well to chemotherapy, may benefit from an operation to remove the part of the lung where the main tumour was situated. This approach to treatment is currently being tested.

RADIOTHERAPY

Treatment with radiotherapy suffers from the same problem as surgery— all too often the tumour has spread outside the area that is being treated. Whilst this is a problem unlikely to be overcome, the development of drugs that can make tumour cells more sensitive to radiation (radio-sensitizers) may mean that radiotherapy will become more useful. Radio-therapy is less able to kill cancer cells that are lacking in oxygen in those parts of the tumour with a poor blood supply, and radiosensitizers are a way of overcoming this problem. The role of radiotherapy together with surgery in localized small-cell lung cancer is currently being tested and the results of these trials will be available in the next few years. Different schedules of radiation (including treatment several times per day) are being tested to see which is most effective. Devices to give radiotherapy inside the main airways have also been developed recently and may be used as an alternative to laser treatment (see p. 80) when an airway is blocked by tumour.

HYPERTHERMIA

Heating all or part of the body may kill some cancer cells. Cells short of oxygen and in an acid environment are particularly sensitive to heat and fortunately these are the very cells most resistant to radiotherapy and chemotherapy (see p. 80). Combinations of these treatments are just starting to be tested and it is hoped that they may be complementary to each other and result in much better killing of cancer cells.

LASER THERAPY

Lasers (with or without porphyrins; see p. 78) may be useful for identify-ing and getting rid of premalignant changes or for treating a tumour that is blocking an airway. Because the treatment only works in parts of the body the laser beam can reach, it is unlikely to be a useful treatment for advanced cases.

Future prospects in lung cancer 109

INTERFERON AND IMMUNOTHERAPY

Interferon is a naturally occurring substance that is normally produced by the body in response to viral infections. It has some anti-cancer effects but these are currently minimal, and it causes unpleasant 'flu-like' symptoms. Despite all the excitement in the media a few years ago, it is not very useful by itself in lung cancer, although it is currently being tested together with chemotherapy. Other substances that work by stimulating the immune system—helping it to fight the cancer—are being looked for but at present none seem very useful.

CHEMOTHERAPY

Drug therapy is now the usual treatment in small-cell lung cancer and can cure a small proportion of people. Most of the rest will benefit from treatment, although there are inevitably side effects from the drugs. Chemotherapy for non-small-cell lung cancer is much more experimental. There is therefore a great need to develop more effective and less toxic drug treatments. Improved understanding of the biology of cancer cells may allow the production of novel drugs that can attack what it is in a cell that makes it cancerous. Drugs that can reverse the process of the development of cancer (transformation) are the goal of much research and may be the answer that scientists and doctors are looking for. However, before such drugs can be developed we need to know more about how normal and cancerous cells work (see Chapter 15).

SYMPTOMATIC CARE

As many people with lung cancer cannot be cured it is very important that the care of symptoms and the support of patients and their family continues to develop. Even if cure is out of the question, much can be done to make patients feel better and to prolong life. For most, an open and honest approach makes things more bearable. The loss of control of all that is happening to them is distressing, and many patients want to be part of their treatment and to help themselves. Because of this, self-help groups have developed in some parts of the country (see p. 120 for details of how to find a self-help group in your area).

The failure of conventional medicine to cure or adequately support some patients with cancer has meant that there has been an increasing interest in alternative approaches. Although these groups often help

110 Lung cancer: the facts

patients, so many 'new' treatments are tried at once that it is difficult to know which, if any, are of any use. The greatest help for most patients seems to come from the emotional support and encouragement they provide. Patients are encouraged to help themselves, which can only be beneficial, but there is no evidence that the diets, enemas, certain drugs (such as laetril) and other treatments can cure cancer.

Although conventional medicine is rightly suspicious of many of the claims of 'alternative cures' it needs to learn more about holistic approaches and about the emotional support of patients. Getting patients involved in their own treatment, helping them to cope with emotional stresses and providing care for the 'whole' patient and their family makes sense.

Lung cancer remains a devastating disease and there is no easy cure-all on the horizon, but steady progress is being made and whilst the cure rate has not improved dramatically, more and more active treatments are being developed. Some patients with localized small-cell lung cancer are being cured with chemotherapy and the further development of drugs, surgery, radiotherapy, hyperthermia, and immunotherapy, etc. is likely to mean that more patients will be cured in the future. However, for the foreseeable future, the most effective way of reducing the toll of lung cancer is its prevention by persuading more people to stop, or never start, smoking.

15
The new biology

Despite improvements in the treatment of lung cancer in the past 20 years there is much to do. During this time there have been exciting new discoveries in the way cells work and, in particular, in the mechanisms that control their division and growth, and we are at last approaching a position where we will be able to test some of these ideas clinically.

One reason for these advances is that we are now able to grow human lung cancers in tissue culture in the laboratory—lung cancers can now be grown in 'test tubes'. This applies to both small-cell lung cancer and the other types lumped together as non-small-cell tumours (see Chapter 1). The characteristics of these various types of lung cancer and variations on these have all been worked out. In general, small-cell lung cancers have properties that they share with other cells in the body concerned with production of hormones or with nerve cells. These properties are generally absent in the non-small-cell tumours.

Similarly, some lung cancers have features (receptors) that suggest that their growth may be influenced by growth factors. These are chemicals produced by cells to regulate their own division, and that of adjacent cells, to produce new cells (Fig. 19). In the past few years a number of these have been identified and their complex chemical structures defined. This means that we are in a position to develop ways of changing the way growth factors may act on cancer cells. Such an approach is in its infancy and may depend on showing that some cancers handle growth factors or produce growth factors that are very different from normal cells. We can already make pure antibodies (the proteins produced by the body to combat infection, etc) that are specific for particular growth factors or their receptor on the cell and that may stop the growth factors working normally. At the moment these are not clinically useful, but similar techniques or chemicals specifically designed to affect the receptors on cancer cells or to mimic growth factors may be developed as an effective treatment in the future.

DNA is a complex molecule that contains a chemical sequence that codes for the way a cell develops and behaves (Fig. 20). Since its basic

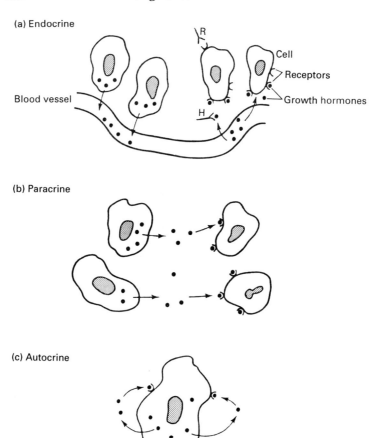

Fig. 19 Stimulation of cell growth by hormones and growth factors. (a) Endocrine stimulation. A hormone is secreted into the bloodstream at one site in the body and is transported to other sites where it interacts with cells that have surface receptors for it. (b) Paracrine stimulation. Cells release a growth factor that interacts with nearby receptor-bearing cells. (c) Autocrine stimulation. A cell releases a growth factor that binds to receptors on its own surface. Antibodies can be produced against the growth hormone itself (Y_H) or against receptors for growth hormones (Y_R).

structure was discovered in the 1950s there has been a rapid increase in our knowledge of DNA and how it works, and this area of understanding has exploded in the past 5–10 years. We now know the genetic code for a

The new biology

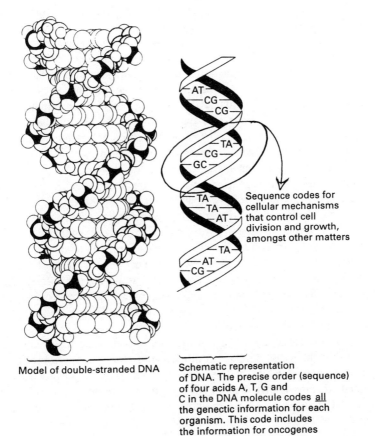

Fig. 20 DNA—the genetic code that controls all aspects of cellular function.

variety of genes that control specific proteins produced by cells and there is a worldwide project to discover the code for all the genes in the human cell—this project of 'mapping the genome' is known as the Human Genome Project.

Recently discoveries have been made about some of the genes in the body concerned with coding for substances that control cell growth and division including, for instance, growth factors. These gene codes were called oncogenes and a large variety of these have been identified, their structure (sequence) has been demonstrated and in many cases the structure of the protein they code for has also been discovered (Fig. 20).

114   Lung cancer: the facts

Study of tissue from lung cancer patients has shown that some tumours contain greater amounts of certain oncogenes than similar normal tissue. This is referred to as amplification, and some tumours have up to 100-fold amplification of particular oncogenes. Studies have shown that patients with such tumours generally have a shorter survival time than those without this amplification, suggesting that cell growth or resistance of the tumour to treatment may be higher when amplification is present. Oncogenes may also appear to be overexpressing themselves and producing more of their effector protein (growth factors, etc) even when they are not present in excess amounts. Minor mutations (changes in their genetic code) may also affect their function.

Studies of how oncogenes, which via their effector proteins, operate to start, speed up, slow down, or stop cell division and growth is a key area of human biology. It is hoped that by understanding these processes we will be able to devise ways of 'turning-off' cancer cells so that they stop growing. Such treatments are not available at present and their use may depend on showing that the growth of cancer cell is, at least partly, dependant on mechanisms that are different from those of normal cells. Minor differences or simple overexpression or amplification of oncogenes and their proteins may make hoped-for treatments difficult to develop, as they will also affect normal cells.

An example of the way growth factors can effect our ability to treat cancer is the recent development of growth factors that control the cells making new blood in the bone marrow. One of the major problems of chemotherapy is that it slows down production of new blood cells and results in anaemia and risk of infection (because of a low level of white cells) or bleeding (because of a low platelet level; platelets are the 'clotting' cells in the blood).

In the last few years we have discovered a series of growth factors that stimulate production of new blood cells (Fig. 21) and these can be manufactured (using genetic engineering techniques) to be given to patients. Treatment with these growth factors definitely reduces the period when patients are at risk from infection (low white cell count) and may allow higher doses of chemotherapeutic drugs to be given. Whether this will make a major impact on cancer treatment is unclear but such techniques are in their infancy and are likely to become increasingly sophisticated as these growth factors are used in combinations and new ones are discovered.

Some genetic conditions predispose certain families to develop cancers. Whilst this is very rarely the case in lung cancer, identification of such

The new biology

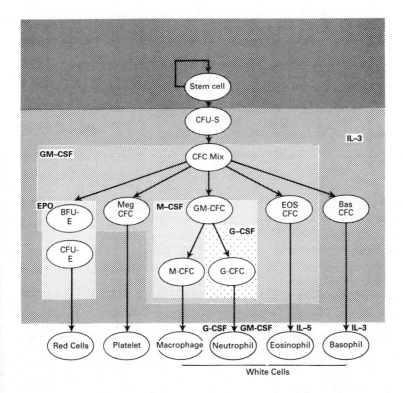

Fig. 21 Schematic representation of the production of new blood cells. Theoretically all the cells are derived from a pool of so-called stem cells. Each cell can, as shown, go down a number of pathways to form red cells, platelets or various types of white cells (bottom line of ovals). Each pathway has a number of steps (the various ovals give the code for the cells involved). Growth factors (see the codes in bold letters) stimulate a particular pathway.

people is very important. It is quite likely that the same gene(s) are affected in normal individuals who are unfortunate enough to become ill with lung cancer and so it would be useful to find which gene(s) are abnormal in these patients. So far, a range of genetic abnormalities has been shown in human lung cancer. One involves loss of part of chromosome 3 (Fig. 22). More recently, a defect has been shown in a gene known as the human retinoblastoma (Rb) gene. This gene determines which family members will develop a cancer of the back of the eye

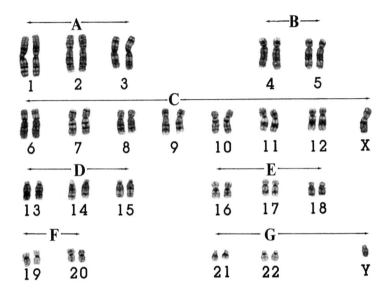

Fig. 22 A normal human male compliment of 46 chromosomes (22 pairs plus one pair of sex chromosomes—the X and Y chromosomes). The chromosomes have been arranged in matching pairs.

(retina); a cancer that shows up very strongly in certain families. This abnormality of the Rb gene is found in 25 per cent of small-cell lung tumours but not in the non-small-cell types. As abnormalities of the Rb gene are also found in a wide range of other common tumours it is likely to have an important role in the biology of cancer.

As well as determining which cells develop into cancer and how they may behave, genes are also involved in the way cancer cells respond to chemotherapy and radiation treatments. In the last 4 years it has become clear that many cells in the body, including cancers, are really remarkably resistant to the drugs and radiation we use to treat cancer. Similarly, some cancers, whilst initially very responsive to treatment, rapidly become totally resistant to a wide variety of drugs. This may be due to cells that were always inherently resistant to treatment continuing to grow and repopulate the tumour or to development (or induction) of resistant cells. Either way, if we know how cells become resistant to treatment we may be able to manipulate this to our advantage.

The new biology 117

This concept of resistance, often called multiple drug resistance, is under active investigation and specific mechanisms of resistance are being found. For instance, a protein that controls how rapidly drugs are actively pumped out of cells (p-glycoprotein) has been found. Cells with high levels of p-glycoprotein may be protected from the effects of drugs as drug levels high enough to kill the cell are never achieved because the cell gets rid of the drug so rapidly. Mechanisms of drug resistance may operate in a wide variety of ways (Table 16) but for them to be potentially useful to us they must either not exist in normal cells or be grossly overexpressed in cancer cells. As with all cancer treatments, a really effective treatment needs to be at least partly specific to the cancer. So far early studies have shown that we *can* manipulate cells that have excess p-glycoprotein, but much work needs to be done. In lung cancer, multiple drug resistance genes have been found in both normal lung tissue and in many lung cancers. Clearly, other similar genes are likely to be found and may offer a more effective target than the p-glycoprotein.

Table 16. Ways in which cells may become resistant to treatment with anti-cancer drugs

Not enough uptake of drug into cells
Activation of the drug is decreased
Deactivation of the drug is increased
Increased use by the cell of salvage mechanisms
Increased repair of DNA damage
Transport out of the cell is increased*

* p-glycoprotein.

This chapter gives only a very brief snapshot of some of the areas of cancer research in progress. There is also much work being done on how and why cells are able to spread and grow in other parts of the body—a process unique to cancer. All these projects rely heavily on our recent understanding of DNA and genes and on new ways of studying and manipulating DNA. The future looks exciting. However, the real key is likely to be difficult to find as effective treatments may need to rely on showing that cancer cells are in some way different from normal cells, or at least different enough to exploit their very differentness.

Further reading

WHAT IS CANCER?

Consumers' Association (1986). *Understanding Cancer*. Consumers' Association, London. ISBN 0340372206.
Looks at the nature and causes of cancer, and various therapies which can be used.

Karol Sikora and Hilary Thomas (1989). *Fight Cancer: how to prevent it and how to fight it*. BBC Books, London. ISBN 0563208481.
A clear book for anybody interested in cancer, its prevention, and its treatment. Good section on complementary care.

Chris Williams (1986). *Cancer: a guide for patients and their families*. Wiley, Chichester. ISBN 0471910171.
A very clear book about cancer and its treatments.

COPING WITH CANCER

Jenny Bryan (1987). *Living with Cancer*. Penguin, Harmondsworth. ISBN 0140094091.
Discusses the facts about cancer and provides advice on how to cope with physical and emotional problems.

Rachael Clyne (1989). *Cancer: your life, your choice*. Thorsons, Wellingborough. ISBN 0722521030.
Book by someone who has close relatives with cancer. Gives an overall help in coping with diagnosis, treatment and caring.

TALKING TO OTHER PEOPLE

Robert Buckman (1988). *I don't know what to say: how to help and support someone who is dying*. Papermac, London. ISBN 0333469836.

Further reading 119

Designed to help the family and friends of those with life-threatening illness, providing practical and emotional guidance.

UNPROVEN/COMPLEMENTARY TREATMENTS

Stephen Fulder (1988). *The handbook of complementary medicine (second edition)*. Oxford University Press. ISBN 0192616900.
Concise review of theoretical, practical, and research aspects of each therapy. Also available in paperback. Includes contact addresses.

Sadhya Rippon (1987). *The Bristol Recipe Book*. Century, London. ISBN 0712615180.
Recipes from the Kitchen Administrator of the Bristol Cancer Help Centre.

Appendix   Sources of help

This section was prepared with the help of 'CancerLink' and is based on their information pack and is used with their permission.

INFORMATION

GENERAL INFORMATION ON CANCER AND HEALTH MATTERS

BACUP
121–3 Charterhouse Street
London
EC1M 6AA
Tel: Information Service 071-608-1661
Counselling Service 071-608-1038
Outside London 0800-181199

Provides information and support to cancer patients and their families and friends. A team of experienced cancer nurses answers telephone calls and written enquiries concerning all aspects of cancer care. Produces a wide range of literature on the main types of cancer and their treatment.

CancerLink
17 Britannia Street
London
WC1X 9JN
Tel: 071-833-2451

CancerLink
9 Castle Terrace
Edinburgh
EH1 2DP
Tel: Edinburgh 031-228-5557

Appendix 121

Provides emotional support and information in response to telephone and letter enquiries on all aspects of cancer from people with cancer, their families and friends and the professionals working with them. Acts as a resource to over 350 cancer support and self help groups throughout Britain; providing information, training, support, and help for people setting up new groups. Produces publications on the emotional and practical aspects of living with cancer.

Cancer Relief Macmillan Fund
Anchor House
15–19 Britten Street
London
SW3 3TZ
Tel: 071-351-7811

Provides care and support for cancer patients and their families in the following ways:

Macmillan nurses are specially trained in pain and symptom control and in the emotional counselling of cancer patients and their relatives. Most of them work in the community with GPs and district nurses caring for patients in their own homes. A smaller number now work in hospitals helping in the care of cancer patients on the wards. The services are a fully integrated part of the NHS.

Cancer Relief has sponsored 14 NHS-run specialist *Macmillan Units*, which provide in-patient wards, home care and day care services for people with advanced cancer.

Patient Grants: Cancer Relief can give immediate help with extra expenses that may not be covered by state benefits e.g. heating costs, bedding, fares, holidays in the UK, home help, nursing, clothing (but not funeral expenses, private treatment, or home improvement). Applications are made by a social worker, health visitor, or community or home care nurse on behalf of the patient, direct to the Patient Grants Department.

Hospice Information Service
St Christopher's Hospice
51–9 Lawrie Park Road
Sydenham
London
SE26 6DZ
Tel: 081-778-9252

122 Lung cancer: the facts

The Hospice Information Service publishes a directory of hospice services providing details of hospices, home care teams, and hospital support teams in the UK and the Republic of Ireland. Copies of the directory are available on receipt of an A5 stamped addressed envelope.

Irish Cancer Society
5 Northumberland Road
Dublin 4
Tel: Dublin 0001-681855
or Freephone 1800-200-300
(in Republic of Ireland only)

Information on all aspects of cancer from nurses via Freephone service. Funds home care and rehabilitation programmes run by voluntary groups for all cancer patients. Support groups for mastectomy, colostomy, and laryngectomy patients, and Hodgkin's disease. Home night-nursing service available on request of patient's doctor or public health nurse.

Tak Tent
Mrs Eileen Smith
National Co-ordinator
4th Floor, G Block
Western Infirmary
Glasgow
G11 6NT
Tel: Glasgow 041-332-2639
or Glasgow 041-357-4519

Information, emotional support, and counselling for cancer patients, relatives, and the professionals who care for them. Support groups, one-to-one counselling and training courses are available.

Tenovus Cancer Information Centre
142 Whitchurch Road
Cardiff
CF4 3NA
Tel: Cardiff 0222-619846

Appendix 123

Provides an education and information service on all aspects of cancer. Primarily concerned with the prevention and early detection of cancers, and with the practical and emotional support necessary for people with cancer and their families. The services provided include an information service, cancer screening mobile clinic providing cervical cancer screening and instructions on breast examination, health education talks, practical advice, and emotional support. They also provide resources and materials.

Ulster Cancer Foundation
Betty McCrum
40-2 Eglantine Avenue
Belfast
BT9 6DX
Tel: 0232-663281/2/3 (office hours)
Helpline: Belfast 0232-663439 (9.30-12.30 weekdays)

Involved in many aspects of cancer, from prevention to patient support. Operates an information helpline for cancer related queries for patients and their families, staffed by experienced cancer nurses who can arrange counselling by personal appointment at the Centre. Rehabilitation support services include: mastectomy advice (volunteer visiting by former patients); laryngectomy club (monthly activities, support in hospitals, and at home); lymphoma support (patient and family link-up); urostomy association (meetings, counselling, home and hospital visiting).

PREVENTION

Action on Smoking & Health (ASH)
5-11 Mortimer Street
London
W1N 7RM
Tel: 071-637-9843

Gives information on the damage smoking does and how to give it up.

124 Lung cancer: the facts

Clinic for Cancer Prevention Advice
6 New Road
Brighton
Sussex
BN1 1VF
Tel: Brighton 0273-727213

Produces publications and brochures on health, lifestyle, and exercise.
Telephone and postal enquiries welcome.

Health Education Authority
Hamilton House
Marbledon Place
London
WC1H 9TX
Tel: 071-383-3833

Information and publications on all aspects of health, including cancer
and cancer prevention.

Health Promotion Authority for Wales
8th Floor
Brunel House
2 Fitzalan Road
Cardiff
CF2 1EB
Tel: Cardiff 0222-472472

Information and publications on all aspects of health, including cancer
and cancer prevention.

Scottish Health Education Group
Health Education Centre
Woodburn House
Canaan Lane
Edinburgh
EH10 4SG
Tel: Edinburgh 031-447-8044
Fax: Edinburgh 031-452-8140

Appendix 125

Information and publications on all aspects of health, including cancer and cancer prevention.

RESEARCH

Cancer Research Campaign (CRC)
2 Carlton House Terrace
London
SW1Y 5AR
Tel: 071-930-8972
Fax: 071-321-0838

CRC funds nationwide research into every aspect of cancer from prevention to cure, from greater understanding of the nature of cancer to education and the psychological support of patients and their families.

Imperial Cancer Research Fund (ICRF)
PO Box 123
Lincolns Inn Fields
London
WC2A 3PX
Tel: 071-242-0200

The Imperial Cancer Research Fund is an independent cancer research institute. It investigates all aspects of the disease including causes, prevention, early diagnosis, and the development of new and improved treatments.

PATIENTS' RIGHTS

Action for Victims of Medical Accidents
Bank Chambers
1 London Road
Forest Hill
London
SE23 3TP
Tel: 081-291-2793

126 Lung cancer: the facts

Works for the fair treatment of victims of medical accidents (those injured by the action or omission of health carers in the course of treatment). Advises victims on their rights, and refers them to solicitors if legal action is possible. Maintains a panel of medical experts who are prepared to give independent opinions, and a panel of experienced solicitors.

Association of Community Health Councils for England and Wales
30 Drayton Park
London
N5 1PB
Tel: 071-609-8405

Community Health Councils are able to make representations to health authorities if they feel that a particular service is not working properly. They welcome general comments from members of the public. Contact the association to find out the Community Health Council in your area.

Patients Association
18 Victoria Park Square
Bethnal Green
London
E2 9PF
Tel: 081-981-5676 or 081-981-5695

Gives advice to individual patients and carers on patients' rights, complaints procedures, and access to health services or appropriate self-help groups. Promotes patients interests nationally to government, professional bodies, and the media. Quarterly newsletter for members; advice leaflets published.

Society for the Prevention of Asbestosis and Industrial Diseases (S.P.A.I.D.)
38 Drapers Lane
Enfield
Middlesex
EN2 8LU
Tel: 0707-873025

Appendix 127

Help for those suffering from, and those working to prevent, industrial diseases. Provides advice on how to make a claim for industrial compensation if someone has cancer which is caused by industrial injury.

COMPLEMENTARY CARE (GENERAL)

Bristol Cancer Help Centre
Grove House
Cornwallis Grove
Clifton
Bristol
BS8 4PG
Tel: Bristol 0272-743216

Offers a holistic healing programme to complement medical treatment, based on a one-day visit to learn about healing, diet, counselling, relaxation, and meditation. Alternatively, the patient can attend a 5 day residential course.

Council for Complementary and Alternative Medicine (CCAM)
38 Mount Pleasant
London
WC1X 0AP
Tel: 071-409-1440

CCAM works to establish educational and ethical standards involved in complementary approaches to health care. It seeks statutory registration and regulation of practitioners for the benefit of the public. The Council can provide information about individual practitioners.

Institute for Complementary Medicine
21 Portland Place
London
W1N 3AF
Tel: 071-636-9543

Can supply referrals from the British Register of Complementary Practitioners. Library available by appointment.

128   Lung cancer: the facts

ACUPUNCTURE

British Acupuncture Association and Register
34 Alderney Street
London
SW1V 4EU
Tel: 071-834-1012 or 071-834-3353

Can supply, for a small fee, a register of members which includes
many trained practitioners with additional medical knowledge and/or
qualifications.

British Medical Acupuncture Society
Newton House
Newton Lane
Whitley
Warrington
WA4 4JA
Tel: Warrington 0925-73727

Promotes the use and understanding of acupuncture as part of the
practice of medicine. Trains qualified doctors and dentists. Publishes a
journal. Membership is available.

'HEALING'

Churches Council for Health and Healing
St Marylebone Parish Church
Marylebone Road
London
NW1 5LT
Tel: 071-486-9644

Puts people in touch with churches in their area involved with the
ministry of Christian healing. A 24-hour answerphone service is
available.

Appendix 129

National Federation of Spiritual Healers
Old Manor Farm Studio
Church Street
Sunbury on Thames
Middlesex
TW16 6RG
Tel: Sunbury 0932 73164

Maintains a list of member healers in all parts of the UK; expect 4 week delay in replies, except in critical cases. Healers are allowed to visit and treat patients in NHS hospitals (must be invited by patients and must not discuss medical treatment).

HERBALISM

British Herbal Medicine Association
Field House
Lye Hole Lane
Redhill
Bristol
Avon
BS18 7TB
Tel: Weston-super-Mare 0934-862994

Aims to protect the interests of users, practitioners, and manufacturers of herbal medicine. Publishes British Herbal Pharmacopoeia. Runs information service, and can refer to local qualified herbal practitioners.

National Institute of Medical Herbalists
Mrs Chacksfields
9 Palace Gate
Exeter
Tel: Exeter 0392-213899

Professional body of herbal practitioners. Provides list of practitioners throughout the country who have all undergone a 4-year training course. Patients are seen on a private basis; fees are charged.

130 Lung cancer: the facts

HOMEOPATHY

'Homeo' is a Greek word meaning 'like' and homeopathy is a system of holistic medicine based on the principle of 'like cures like'. The concept that the body is able to heal itself if its own healing power is correctly stimulated is fundamental to homeopathy. This is achieved by giving certain remedies, derived from plant, mineral, or animal sources. They are prepared and diluted so that tiny amounts of the original substance remain. The preparation process produces energy which stimulates the body's immune system when the remedy, which is often in the form of a pill, is taken.

British Homeopathic Association
27a Devonshire Street
London
W1N 1RJ
Tel: 071-935-2163

The association has a list of all homeopathic doctors and hospitals throughout the UK and has a lending library for members. Publishes a bi-monthly journal and has leaflets on homeopathy.

NATUROPATHY AND OSTEOPATHY

British College of Naturopathy and Osteopathy
General Council and Register of Naturopathy
Frazer House
6 Netherall Gardens
London
NW3 5RR
Tel: 071-435-8728

Can refer callers to local therapists. They produce a national register which costs £1.50 plus SAE. The college also runs a clinic at the above address.

Appendix 131

REFLEXOLOGY

The British School of Reflexology
2 Sheering Road
Old Harlow
Essex
CM17 0LT
Tel: 0279-29060

Please write for information. Can provide information about reflexology, local contacts, and qualified therapists.

RELAXATION

Relaxation for Living
29 Burwood Park Road
Walton on Thames
Surrey
KT12 5LH

Promotes the teaching of physical relaxation. Holds small group classes around the UK, and runs a correspondence course for relaxation teachers.

EMOTIONAL SUPPORT

GENERAL CANCER COUNSELLING

The emotional impact that the diagnosis and treatment of cancer can have on the individual, their families, and friends is well known. Counselling on a one-to-one basis can be a useful tool in helping a person develop their own way of coping with their particular situation. When a person consults a counsellor they won't be told how to cope; rather they will be encouraged to find their own answers. A counsellor is trained to listen, and to try to enable the person to see their situation as it is and to work through their feelings about it. Cancer, along with other chronic life-threatening illnesses, raises particular issues of its own and some counsellors specialize in this field.

132 Lung cancer: the facts

The Association of Black Counsellors
c/o Ms Nicholas
7 Mead Close
Harrow Weald
Middlesex

Aims to enhance the psychological wellbeing of black people and to train black people in counselling skills.

BACUP
121-3 Charterhouse Street
London
EC1M 6AA
Tel: 071-608-1038

Offers a short term counselling service based in their London office.

Bristol Cancer Help Centre
Grove House
Cornwallis Grove
Clifton
Bristol
Tel: Bristol 0272-743216

A team of counsellors experienced in working with people with cancer.

The British Association for Counselling
1 Regent Place
Rugby
CV21 2PJ
Tel: Rugby 0788-578328

Produces a directory of organizations and individual counsellors in the UK.

Appendix 133

Counselling Information Scotland
Scottish Health Education Group
Woodburn House
Cannon Lane
Edinburgh
EH10 4SG
Tel: Edinburgh 031-452-8989

Can provide information on counsellors in Scotland.

The Westminster Pastoral Foundation
23 Kensington Square
London
W8 5HN
Tel: 081-937-6956

Offer specific counselling for people with serious physical illness.

Other professionals are available to offer emotional support; for example, Macmillan nurses aim to offer emotional support for cancer patients and their families. They can visit people in their homes. A GP can arrange for one to call if there is a local service.

SELF-HELP GROUPS

These are too numerous to list here, but CancerLink and BACUP may be able to help find such a group in your area. Their addresses and telephone numbers are on page 120.

BEREAVEMENT

When considering the needs of the bereaved person, support is sought from the community, from family, friends, and neighbours. If the bereaved person is well-supported by people who understand and acknowledge the need for grief and accept it as a process that may go on for some time, then they may not need much more support from other sources. Difficulties often begin to occur where such support is absent. If, for example,

134 Lung cancer: the facts

they have no close friends nearby, support can be withdrawn too soon or the bereaved person has felt too awkward about asking for help because they feel they 'should have got over it'. Sometimes the circumstances surrounding the death may indicate the need for more support.

People who have not had a major bereavement tend to underestimate the time it takes to work through feelings of loss and grief. Difficulties may be experienced, in the normal course of events, for at least two years. It may be that the local cancer self-help group can offer the bereaved person the support they need. You may want to refer them to a specialist group or individual. There will be occasions when more support will be needed, and this support may come in the form of a bereavement support group or individual one-to-one counselling.

Compassionate Friends
6 Denmark Hill
Bristol
BS1 5DQ
Tel: Bristol 0272-292778

A nationwide self-help organization of parents who offer support and help for those parents who have lost a child of any age (including adult) who have died through any cause, by others similarly bereaved. Personal and group support through befriending, not counselling. They provide a quarterly newsletter, postal library, and a range of leaflets.

Cruse Bereavement Care
Cruse House
126 Sheen Road
Richmond
Surrey
TW9 0UR
Tel: 081-940-4818

Runs a counselling service for all bereaved people throughout the UK, offering understanding, practical advice, and information.

Foundation for Black Bereaved Families
Lorreene Hunte
11 Kingston Square

Appendix 135

Salters Hill
London
SE19 1JE
Tel: 081-761-7228

Help and support for bereaved black people of African and Caribbean origins. They offer counselling, financial advice, home visits, and attend funerals.

Gay Bereavement Project
Unitarian Rooms
Hoop Lane
London
NW11 8DS
Tel: 081-455-8894 (7.00pm–Midnight)

A telephone helpline for people bereaved by the death of a same-sex partner.

National Association of Bereavement Services
122 Whitechapel High Street
London
E1 7PT
Tel: 071-247-1080 (referrals requests)
      071-247-0671 (admin.)

Set up in 1988 to co-ordinate the many unsupported and often isolated bereavement services. The Association's aims include compiling a National Register of existing services.

FINANCIAL SOURCES

ACCIDENTS AND SERIOUS ILLNESS AT WORK

If someone has suffered an accident or serious illness because of their work there are a number of non-contributory benefits which may be

136   Lung cancer: the facts

relevant. To find out more get leaflets N16 and NI10 (from your local DSS, post office or advice agency).

If someone is unable to work because of cancer which has been caused by industrial injury they are entitled to Sickness or Invalidity benefit even if they have not paid the correct National Insurance contributions. They may also make a claim for industrial compensation. Advice on how and when to go about this is available from:

Society for the Prevention of Asbestosis and Industrial Diseases
38 Drapers Road
Enfield
Middlesex
EN2 8LU
Tel: 0707-873025

If they are a member of a Trade Union there may be a benevolent fund available.

CARERS

People may be entitled to the following help from the DSS:

- Invalid Care Allowance if they are looking after someone who needs help and support for at least 35 hours a week and is also receiving Attendance Allowance. See leaflet NI212.
- Income Support and other means-tested benefits.
- Help from the Social Fund.
- National Insurance credits to protect their pension entitlement.

Attendance Allowance

Attendance Allowance is a non-contributory benefit payable to someone who needs a lot of looking after. Attendance Allowance is paid at two rates—the lower rate is paid if a person needs attention during the day or night but not both; the higher rate is paid if the attention is needed both night and day. A person must normally have satisfied the conditions for getting the benefits for six months before they get Attendance Allowance. Anyone who is terminally ill can claim Attendance Allowance of £41.65 per week without having to wait for the 6 month qualifying

Appendix 137

period. In Social Security law, 'terminally ill' means that a person has a progressive disease with a reasonable expectation of life of six months or less.

To find out more get leaflet DS2 from the DSS or Citizens' Advice Bureau.

PRESCRIPTION SEASON TICKETS

These are properly called prepayment certificates and work like a season ticket. They can work out cheaper for people who need a lot of prescriptions but aren't eligible for exemption from charges. They can be bought by completing Form FP94, which is available from the DSS, post office, chemist, or the Family Practitioner Committee and should be returned to the Family Practitioner Committee, whose address is in the telephone book.

If someone has already paid charges and wants to apply for a refund ask a chemist for form FP57. There is a 3 month time limit for claiming a refund.

For details of NHS prescription charges and exemptions get leaflet P11 (from your local DSS, post office, or advice agency).

INSURANCE

People may be worried that they will be refused insurance because of their health situation. It may be useful to suggest a listed broker who can shop around for the best policy. People should check that the person selling financial products or services is fully authorized. FIMBRA (Financial Intermediaries Managers and Brokers Regulatory Association) members must give independent financial advice best suited to the person's needs. A list of local financial advisors should be available from local banks, building societies or contact the

Campaign for Independent Financial Advice
Telephone 081-200-3000

Holiday Care Service
2 Old Bank Chambers
Station Road

Horley
Surrey
RH6 9HW
Tel: 0923-774535

Radar
25 Mortimer Street
London
W1N 8AB
Tel: 071-637-5400

Produce information factsheets on holiday insurance cover. The Holiday Care Service has their own travel insurance service.

LAUNDRY

Help toward laundry costs may be met from Social Security as a special need (see Social Security Benefits section).

CHARITIES PROVIDING FINANCIAL HELP

Cancer Relief Macmillan Fund
15/19 Britten Street
London
SW3 3TZ
Tel: 071-351-7811

Provides financial help through grants towards the cost of services and goods such as travel, home-nursing, fuel costs, and child-minding fees. Applications should be made through community nurses or social workers.

Marie Curie Cancer Care
28 Belgrave Square
London
SW1X 8QG
Tel: 071-235-3325

Appendix 139

Welfare grant schemes available; applications should be made through the district nursing service.

PRACTICAL HELP

SITTING SERVICE

A 'sitter' is someone who will come and 'sit' with a person at home, giving the person who normally cares for them a break. The kind of help organizations offer varies; some will keep the person company but will not carry out any personal household tasks, others may prepare a meal or get the person up, and wash and dress them. These schemes may be run by Social Services Departments or voluntary organizations. Contact the Social Services or the local Council for Voluntary Service.

CARE ATTENDANT SCHEMES

The aim of these schemes is to provide relief for carers. Care Attendants usually do everything that a carer would do. They are trained and employed by the scheme. They are not meant to replace other services such as Home Helps or District Nurses. Schemes may be provided by Health Authorities, Local Authorities or voluntary organizations. These include Home Care Attendant Schemes, Extended Home Help Schemes, and Crossroads Care Attendant Schemes. For local provision check with the Social Services department and the local Council for Voluntary Service.

Crossroads Care
10 Regent Place
Rugby
Warwickshire
CV21 2PN
Tel: 0788-73653

This is the largest network of voluntary projects. There are around 150 schemes all over the UK. For details of local contacts check with the above address.

140 Lung cancer: the facts

The United Kingdom Home Care Association
c/o Care Alternatives Limited
206 Worple Road
Wimbledon
London
SW20 8PN
Tel: 081-946-8202

This is an association of private home care providers aiming to set codes and standards of practice.

Private agencies also offer a home care service. Fees vary, so it is important to check out how much hiring a private sitter or care attendant will cost.

Leaflets The following organizations produce leaflets that may be useful regarding help in the home:

Age Concern
Astral House
1268 London Road
London
SW16 4ER
Tel: 081-679-8000

Produce a leaflet called *Companions and Help at Home*. For a copy send large SAE and ask for Factsheet 6.

Counsel and Care for the Elderly
Tyman House
16 Bonny Street
London
NW1 9PG
Tel: 071-485-1566

Produce a leaflet *Help at Home*. For a copy send a large SAE requesting Factsheet 9.

Appendix 141

MAKING A WILL

If you are supporting someone who is dying they may want some information about how to sort out their affairs and what arrangements they might need to make, such as how to make a will.

Anyone over 18 can make a will. Wills do not have to be drawn up by solicitors; pre-printed forms are available from stationers. It is very important that someone drawing up a will does it properly.

There are books to guide people (e.g. *Wills and Probate*, published by Which? Books) and the local Citizens Advice Bureau may also be able to advise.

It can cost around £50 for a solicitor to draw up a will. If a person is on Income Support and does not have savings above a certain level they are entitled to two hours of free advice from a solicitor who is in the Legal Aid scheme. If they are on a low income, but not on Income Support, they may be able to get two hours of advice for a reduced fee. Again, the Citizens Advice Bureau will be able to give more information.

Age Concern
Astral House
1268 London Road
London
SW16 4ER
Tel: 081-679-8000

Have produced a form that a person can complete which contains information that would enable the next of kin or executors to establish that person's wishes and the whereabouts of important documents. The leaflet is called *Instructions for my next of kin and executors upon my death*. For a copy send SAE.

Glossary

ACTH: adrenocorticotrophic hormone. Stimulates the production of hormones from the adrenal gland.

Adenocarcinoma: tumour of the glands.

Adrenal glands: glands on the kidney that secrete hormones.

Anaemia: lack of red blood cells.

Antibody: substance produced by the body to fight infection.

Aspirate: to withdraw fluid.

Aspirin: a common painkiller.

Biopsy: removal of tissue or fluid for examination under a microscope.

Bronchi: the trachea divides into two tubes (the bronchi). One goes into each lung.

Bronchitis: inflammation of the bronchi.

Bronchoscope: an instrument inserted down the trachea so that the doctor can see inside the bronchi.

Bronchoscopy: the technique of using a bronchoscope.

Cancer: a general term for growths in the body. Cancers tend to cause destruction of nearby tissues, spread to other parts of the body and to recur after removal.

Cancer in situ: a small tumour that has not spread from its original site.

Carcinogen: a substance that promotes cancer.

Carcinoma: a malignant growth of epithelial tissue like the skin and glands.

Chemotherapy: treatment using drugs.

Chromosome: the genetic material found in every cell in the body. Every human cell contains 46 chromosomes, which carry the genes.

Combination chemotherapy: treatment with a combination of drugs.

Corticosteroid: steroid hormones produced by the adrenal glands.

Cytology: examination of individual cells under the microscope.

Dose-response effect: the effect of different doses on the response to a treatment.

Dysplasia: development of abnormal tissue.

Electron microscope: a very high resolution microscope.

Emphysema: damage to the lungs caused by loss of fine air pockets (alveoli).

Excision: removal by cutting-out.

Gene: a chemical structure on the chromosome that is responsible for passing on hereditary information.

Haemoptysis: coughing up blood.

Hormone: a chemical secreted into the bloodstream that controls the functioning of the rest of the body.

Glossary 143

Hyperthermia: very high body temperature.

Immunotherapy: treatment that uses the body's immune system to fight the cancer.

Inflammation: reaction of tissues to infection. Characterized by pain, swelling, redness and heat.

Isotope: a chemical that can exist in two physical forms. Radioactive isotopes are used in medical research because their position can be monitored.

Large-cell cancer: type of cancer found in smokers. May develop in the central or peripheral parts of the lungs. Can spread to the airways, lymph glands and to other parts of the body in the bloodstream.

Larynx: the voice box.

Laser: light amplification by Stimulated Emission of Radiation. Energy transmitted as heat that can destroy cells.

Latent period: period between exposure to a carcinogen and development of cancer.

Lobectomy: excision of a lobe.

Localized disease: disease confined to one part of the body.

Malaise: discomfort.

Malignant: dangerous, fatal.

Mesothelioma: tumour of the lining of the lung. It is associated with exposure to asbestos.

Metaplasia: transformation of one type of cell into a different type.

Metastasis: the transference of disease from one part of the body to another.

Metastasize: the process of metastasis.

Metastatic: a tumour that has the ability to metastasize.

Monoclonal antibody: strain of antibody that can be used to differentiate tumours.

Mortality: the death rate.

Mucosa: a membrane/lining that contains glands.

Nausea: sickness.

Oedema: swelling of tissue caused by fluid.

Oesophagus: the gullet.

Oncogene: gene capable of stimulating the formation of a tumour.

Paraneoplastic: disease associated with malignancy but that is not directly caused by the tumour.

Paroxysm: a sudden attack.

Passive smoking: inhalation of other peoples' cigarette smoke.

Pericardial: referring to the sac that surrounds the heart.

Phototherapy: treatment by exposure to artificial blue light.

Placebo: a harmless, inert substance that looks identical to the substance being tested.

Pleura: membrane lining the lungs.

Pleural effusion: fluid in the space between the lung and the chest wall.

Pleuritic pain: pain in the lining of the lungs.

144 Lung cancer: the facts

Pneumonectomy: removal of a lung.

Precancerous: changes that occur before a cancer forms. They usually result in cancer.

Prophylactic: preventive.

Radiotherapy: treatment by X-rays.

Remission: period when the cancer has reduced in size or disappeared.

Resection: surgical removal (excision).

Sarcoma: malignant growth of bone and muscle.

Secondary tumour: metastasis of a tumour from another part of the body.

Squamous lung cancer: common in smokers. Cancerous cells develop in the airways.

Steroid: naturally occurring group of hormones.

Thoracotomy: surgical exposure of the chest cavity.

TNM system: Tissue, Node, Metastasis system of grading cancers.

Trachea: the windpipe.

Tumour: a mass of abnormal tissue that resembles normal tissue but that serves no useful purpose. May be benign (does not infiltrate nearby tissue or cause metastases; unlikely to recur if removed) or malignant.

Ultrasound: a technique for visualizing inner structures of the body by analysing the echoes of very high-pitched sound.

Index

acanthosis nigricans 33
ACTH 87
acupuncture 25, 96, 128
adenocarcinoma of lung 6, 7, 49, 57
air pollution 20
airways obstruction 32
alkaline phosphatase 44
alternative (complementary) treatments
   109-10, 127-31
antibodies
   monoclonal 9
   tumour cells 107
antidiuretic hormone (ADH), excess
   87-8
appetite, loss of 59, 69, 96-7
asbestos 12, 13, 74, 76
attendance allowance 136-7
aversion therapy 25

BACUP 120, 132
barium swallow 42
BCG therapy 65-6, 70
bereavement 133-5
biology, new 111-17
biopsy
   lung tissue 36
   lymph node 34
   pleural 35
blood cell production 114, 115
blood tests 44
blood vessels, diseases of 21-2
bone marrow
   examination 44
   transplantation 73
bones
   changes 33
   metastatic spread to 34, 43-4, 88-9
brain
   generalized effects on 91
   metastatic spread to 34, 44-5, 70-1,
      89-90
   radiotherapy 71, 89, 90

breathlessness 32
bronchial gland tumours 77
bronchioloalveolar carcinoma 7
bronchitis 22-3
bronchoscopy 35, 40

cachexia 97
calcium excess (hypercalcaemia) 88
cancer 3-4
   counselling 131-3
   further reading 118-19
   related to smoking 21
CancerLink 120-1
Cancer Relief Macmillan Fund 121, 138
carcinoid tumours 8, 76
carcinosarcomas 77
cardiovascular diseases 21-2
care attendant schemes 139-40
carers 136-7
chemotherapy (anti-cancer drug therapy)
   combination 62-4
   combined with surgery/radiotherapy
      63, 64, 65, 70
   future outlook 66, 109
   mesothelioma 75-6
   non-small-cell lung cancer 61-4
   resistance of cancer cells to 116-17
   side-effects 69, 114
   small-cell lung cancer 67-9
   symptomatic care 82, 84
chest discomfort/pain 31-2
chest drains (tubes) 54, 55, 85
chest infections 32, 82
chest X-rays 34, 40
clinical trials 103-5
clubbing 33, 89
complementary (alternative) care
   109-10, 127-31
computed tomography (CT scans) 40,
   43, 44, 45
concentration, loss of 59, 71
consent, informed 103-4

Index

coronary heart disease 21-2
corticosteroid (cortisol) excess 87
Corynebacterium parvum therapy 70
cough 29-31, 59, 92-3
counselling, cancer 131-3
cylindroma 77

depression 95
dermatomyositis 33, 92
dexamethasone 90, 97
DNA 111-13
drug resistance genes 116-17
drug therapy
anti-cancer, *see* chemotherapy
stopping smoking 25
see also steroid therapy

electrical stimulation, peripheral nerves
96
electron microscopy 9
emotional support 131-5
emphysema 22-3
empyema 56
exploratory operations 36, 52

families, cancer-prone 12-13, 114-16
financial sources 135-9
food supplements 97
fractures 89
frozen sections 54

gallium-67 isotope test 41-2
genetic factors, link between smoking
and lung cancer 20-1
genetics 113-17
grade, tumour 8-9
group therapy 25
growth factors 73, 111, 112, 113-14,
115

haematoporphyrins 78, 79
haemoptysis 30-1
hair loss 69, 71
'healing' 128-9
heart disease 21-2
heat treatment (hyperthermia) 73, 80-1,
108
helpful organizations 27, 100, 120-41

herbalism 129
hoarseness 32, 91
Hodgkin's disease 77
homeopathy 130
hormones
production by cancer cells 9, 33, 86-8
stimulation of cell growth 112
Horner's syndrome 91
Hospice Information Service 121-2
hypercalcaemia 88
hyperthermia 73, 80-1, 108
hypertrophic pulmonary osteoarthropathy
33, 89
hypnosis 25, 96

immunotherapy 65-6, 70, 109
infections
chest 32, 82
susceptibility to 69
information sources 120-31
informed consent 103-4
insurance 137-8
interferon 66, 70, 109
interleukin-2 66, 70
isotope scanning 41-2, 43

large-cell lung cancer 6, 7, 49, 57
laser surgery 79
laser therapy 78-80, 82-3, 108
laundry 138
levamisole 66, 70
liver metastases 34, 42-3
lobectomy 54
lung cancer
causes 14-23
development 4-5
diagnosis 29-37, 99
distant spread and metabolic effects 33
early diagnosis and screening 36-7,
106-7
future prospects 106-10
grade 8-9
people at risk 10-13
prevention 106, 123-5
secondary or metastatic spread 33-4
staging tests 38-45, 99, 107
symptoms 29-32
talking about 98-100
tests used in diagnosis 34-6
treatment, *see* treatment
types 6

Index

147

lung collapse 82-3
lung function tests 50
lung tissue, aspiration 36
lung tumours
 rare 76-7
 secondary (metastases) 77
lymph nodes
 biopsy 34
 tumour spread to 33, 36, 40-2
lymphomas (lymph gland tumours) 77

magnetic resonance imaging (MRI) 44-5
mediastinoscopy 40, 41
mediastinotomy 41, 42
memory, loss of 59, 71
men, lung cancer deaths 10-12
mesothelioma 6, 8, 74-6
metastatic disease 33-4, 42-5
mixed tumours 77
monoclonal antibodies 9

narcotic drugs 94-5
naturopathy 130
nausea 59
nerve blocks 95-6
nerves, lung cancer spread to 91
nervous system disorders 33, 89-91
new biology 111-17
nicotine chewing gum 25
non-small-cell lung cancer 6, 111
 combined therapy 64-5
 immunotherapy 65-6
 inoperable tumours 57-66
 staging 39-45
 surgery 49-57, 107
 treatment 49-66, 107

occupational risks 12, 13, 20, 74
oncogenes 9, 113-14
osteoarthropathy, hypertrophic
   pulmonary 33, 89
osteopathy 130
oxygen therapy 54-6

pain
 bone 88-9
 chest 31-2
 control 93-6
 postoperative 55
 on swallowing 59

pain-killers 93-5
patients' rights 125-7
pericardial effusion 32, 86
peripheral nerve stimulation 96
peritoneum 76
p-glycoprotein 117
photoradiation 78-9
phototherapy 73, 79
physiotherapy 55
placebo therapy 25
pleura 76
 biopsy 35
pleural effusions 32, 35, 84-5
pleurocentesis 85
pneumonectomy 53, 54
pneumothorax 36, 85
postoperative care 54-5
practical help 139-41
precancerous (premalignant) changes
   4-5, 79
prednisone 97
pregnancy, smoking in 23
prescription season tickets 137
prevention 106, 123-5
pulmonary blastomas 77

radiosensitizers 66, 108
radiotherapy
 brain 71, 89, 90
 combined with chemotherapy 70
 combined with surgery 64-5
 effectiveness 60-1
 future outlook 66, 108
 inoperable non-small-cell lung cancer
   58-61
 internal 80, 83, 108
 mesothelioma 75
 side-effects 59-60
 small-cell lung cancer 69-70
 symptomatic care 82, 83, 89, 90
radon gas 13
reflexology 131
rehabilitation 55
relaxation 131
research, information sources 125
retinoblastoma (Rb) gene 115-16

sarcomas 77
screening, lung cancer 36, 106-7
segmentectomy 54
self-help groups 133

148 Index

sitting service 139
skeletal survey 43-4
skin, reddening and soreness 59
skin rashes 33, 92
sleepiness 59, 71
small-cell lung cancer 6, 8, 111
 outlook 72-3
 spread to brain 89
 staging 38, 45
 treatment 67-73, 107-8
smoking 15-19, 74, 106
 health hazards 21-3
 link with lung cancer 15-19
  effect of stopping smoking 18-19
  genetic influences 20-1
  investigations 16-18
 passive 19
 precancerous changes and 79
 in pregnancy 23
 reasons for starting 27-8
 stopping 24-8
spinal cord, lung cancer spread to 90
sputum cytology 34
squamous lung cancer 6, 7
 development 4-5
 results of surgery 57
 treatment 49
staging tests 38-45, 99, 107
steroid hormones, excess production 87
steroid therapy 84, 90, 92, 97
superior sulcus tumours 64-5, 91
superior vena caval obstruction 32,
  83-4
support organizations 27, 100, 120-41
surgery 49-57
 combined with chemotherapy/
  radiotherapy 63, 64-5
 exploratory operations 36, 52
 future outlook 66, 107-8
 laser 79
 mesothelioma 75
 possible complications 56
 postoperative care 54-5
 procedures 51-4
 rehabilitation after 55
 results 56-7

selection of patients for 49-50, 51
 small-cell lung cancer 70
swallowing, painful 59
symptomatic care 82-97, 109-10

Tenovus Cancer Information Centre
  122-3
thoracotomy 54
tiredness 59, 69
TNM staging system 39
tracheal cancer 77
treatment 47
 alternative (complementary) 109-10,
  127-31
 future prospects 107-10
 mesothelioma 75-6
 non-small-cell lung cancer 49-66, 107
 rare lung tumours 76-7
 small-cell lung cancer 67-73, 107-8
 symptomatic 82-97, 109-10

ultrasound 43

venous obstruction 83-4
venous thrombosis, deep 56
ventilation, mechanical 55
vitamin A deficiency 20
vocal cord damage 32, 91

weight loss 96-7
will, making a 141
women
 lung cancer deaths 10-12
 smoking by 28
work
 accidents and serious illness 135-6
 exposure to carcinogens 12, 13, 74

X-rays
 chest 34, 40
 skeletal survey 43-4